PLANNED PARENTHOOD IN EUROPE
A Human Rights Perspective

PLANNED PARENTHOOD IN EUROPE

A Human Rights Perspective

Edited by
PHILIP MEREDITH and LYN THOMAS

on behalf of the International Planned
Parenthood Federation, Europe Region

CROOM HELM
London ● Sydney ● Dover, New Hampshire

©1986 International Planned Parenthood Federation Europe Region
Croom Helm Ltd, Provident House, Burrell Row,
Beckenham, Kent BR3 1AT

Croom Helm Australia Pty Ltd, Suite 4, 6th Floor,
64-76 Kippax Street, Surry Hills, NSW 2010, Australia

British Library Cataloguing in Publication Data

Planned parenthood in Europe: a human rights
   perspective.
   1. Birth control — Europe
   I. Meredith, Philip   II. Thomas, Lyn
   304.6'66'094   HQ766.5.E87
   ISBN 0-7099-1331-1

Croom Helm, 51 Washington Street, Dover,
New Hampshire 03820, USA

Library of Congress Cataloging in Publication Data
Main entry under title:

Planned parenthood in Europe.

   Includes index.
   1. Birth control—law and legislation—Europe.
2. Birth control—Europe. 3. Family size—Europe.
I. Meredith, Philip, 1950– . II. Thomas,
Lyn, 1950– . III. International planned parenthood
federation. Europe region. (DNLM: 1. Community
health services—Europe. 2. Family planning—Europe.
HQ 766.5.E9)
KJ3575.P58   1986   304.6'6'094   85-26888
ISBN 0-7099-1331-1

Printed and bound in Great Britain
by Billing & Sons Limited, Worcester.

CONTENTS

Chapter Six:
COUNTRY CASE STUDIES

Chapter Seven:
CONCLUSION

APPENDICES

BIBLIOGRAPHY

INDEX

The **International Planned Parenthood Federation** is the world's leading voluntary family planning organisation. It is a federation of independent family planning (or planned parenthood) associations (PPAs) with members in 119 countries. Founded in 1952, its aims are: to initiate and support family planning services throughout the world, and to increase understanding by people and governments of the interrelated issues of population, resources, environment and development.

Europe is one of the six Regions of the IPPF, consisting of 21 national PPAs, which share common interests in promoting planned parenthood.

*****

In 1980, the Yugoslav PPA delegates to the IPPF Europe Regional Council proposed a project to inquire into 'the status of planned parenthood as an integral part of human rights, and into the conditions for the implementation of these human rights, on the basis of IPPF, United Nations and other declarations on this subject'.

Produced with the assistance of PPA volunteers and staff in 18 countries, this report comprises the most detailed examination yet undertaken of the current status of planned parenthood-related laws <u>and</u> the services to which they refer. Using a review of international declarations on planned parenthood as a human right (1946-84) as evidence of the general commitment of governments, the report presents data which identifies the degree of specific commitment to this right in terms of states' involvement in the provision of the <u>means</u> for their citizens to exercise it.

However, it is neither presumed that governments should take all responsibility for the realisation of such rights, nor that legislation is the only or necessary means to achieve this situation. Rather, the report is concerned with the merits and demerits of actual/potential state involvement in planned parenthood from the standpoint of the PPA. This is not, therefore, a vehicle for IPPF recommendations but an aid to PPAs in developing relations with their own governments, making use of an international comparison of situations confronting sister Associations.

The project's findings, and the human rights premises on which they are based, formed the agenda of a discussion between selected government and PPA participants in December 1984. This seminar, which was held by the IPPF Europe Region with the aim of furthering the dialogue and working relationship between PPAs and their national governments, is summarised in the conclusion of this report.

Jürgen Heinrichs
Regional President
London, March 1985

PROJECT ORGANISATION

Regional Working Group

Marie-France Coulet
Mouvement Français pour le Planning Familial, Paris.   (PPA)

Freddy Deven
Centrum voor Bevolkings- en Gezinsstudiën (CBGS), Brussels.

Mikolaj Kozakiewicz
Academy of Sciences, Warsaw.

Nevenka Petric
Family Planning Council of Yugoslavia, Belgrade.   (PPA)

Thorsten Sjövall
Riksförbundet för Sexuell Upplysning, Stockholm.   (PPA)

Regional Bureau:

Julian Heddy
Philip Meredith
Lyn Thomas

The data supplied by PPA contact persons in 19 countries is gratefully acknowledged.

The Regional Working Group would also like to thank Lenore Kupperstein and Nuray Finçancioglü of the IPPF Policy Department for their contributions to sections of this report.

Österreichische Gesellschaft für Familienplanung
Universitätsfrauenklinik II
Spitalgasse 23
A1090 VIENNA
Austria

Centra Gezinsplanning en Seksuele Opvoeding/
Fédération Belge pour le Planning Familial
Troonstraat 51
1050 BRUSSELS
Belgium

Family Development Council
Institute of Obstetrics & Gynaecology
2 Zdrave Street
SOFIA 1431
Bulgaria

Family Planning Association of Cyprus
Boumboulina Street 25
NICOSIA
Cyprus

Foreningen for Familieplanlaegning
Aureh jvej 2
2900 HELLERUP
Denmark

Väestöliitto
Kalevankatu 16
00100 HELSINKI 10
Finland

Mouvement Français pour le Planning Familial
4 Square St Irénée
75011 PARIS
France

Ehe und Familie
Leninalle 70
25 ROSTOCK
German Democratic Republic

Pro Familia
Cronstettenstraße 30
6 FRANKFURT/MAIN 1
Federal Republic of Germany

Hungarian Scientific Society for Family & Women's Welfare
Buday Laszlo u 1-3
1024 BUDAPEST
Hungary

Irish Family Planning Association
15 Mountjoy Square
DUBLIN 1
Ireland

Unione Italiana Centri de Educazione Matrimoniale e
Prematrimoniale
Via Eugenio Chiesa 1
20122 MILAN
Italy

Mouvement Luxembourgeois pour le Planning Familial et
l'Education Sexuelle
18-20 Rue Glesener
LUXEMBOURG
Luxembourg GD

J Rutgers Stichting
Groot Hertoginnelaan 201
THE HAGUE
Netherlands

Norsk Forening for Familieplanlegging
c/o Kari Kromann
Department of Social Medicine
Rikshospitalet
Pilestredet 32
OSLO 1
Norway

Towarzystwo Rozwoju Rodziny
U1 Karowa 31
WARSAW
Poland

Associaçao para o Planeamento da Familia
Rua Artilharia Um 38-2° DT°
LISBON 1200
Portugal

Riksförbundet för Sexuell Upplysning
Rosenlundsgatan 13
STOCKHOLM 17
Sweden

Türkiye Aile Plânlamasi Dernegi
Ataç Sokak 73/3
ANKARA
Turkey

Family Planning Association
27-35 Mortimer Street
LONDON W1N 7RJ
United Kingdom

Family Planning Council of Yugoslavia
Bulevar Lenjina 6
11070 BELGRADE
Yugoslavia

Chapter One

INTRODUCTION

The IPPF in general, and the Europe Region in particular, have worked for many years to ensure that international resolutions codifying basic human rights include reference to the right of individuals to decide (without external pressure) on the number and spacing of their children. Such efforts have not been without success. Since 1948, when the General Assembly of the United Nations adopted and proclaimed a Universal Declaration of Human Rights, the inclusion of 'planned parenthood' - defined as the unfettered right of an individual or couple to decide on the number and spacing of their children (including the decision to remain childless) - has been supported by different UN bodies and in Council of Europe Resolutions.

In real terms, what is implied by the notion of a human 'right' to decide on the number and spacing of children is the extent to which individuals have access to the knowledge and the practical means to regulate their fertility. Therefore, access to contraceptive knowledge, methods and services lies at the heart of this right. However, the implications of this right go further than this. For access to fertility regulation confers on the individual the means of a freer expression of sexuality itself. Attaining the means of control over such biological processes is a core component of women's rights and sexual liberation.

The declarations of international bodies on the subject of basic rights to planned parenthood have, in many respects, been reflected in the gradual legal or constitutional codification of such rights by European national governments. Thus, Simons was able to state that:

> A transformation has occurred over the past two decades in the policies of European governments towards the provision of assistance with contraception.(1)

Reviewing the situation as it was in 1965, he reported that there was little active government support of contraceptive services. In fact legal restrictions on their provision existed in a large number of European countries. However, to differing degrees, both in the Eastern and Western European states, so-called 'modern' or technical/medical methods of contraception have become increasingly available, partly as a result of the commitment of these states to planned parenthood rights as defined by international declarations.(2)

In spite of this, for many people in Europe, unhindered access to information and the means of fertility regulation as a human right has yet to be realised. Significant gaps remain between the formal acceptance by governments of the principle of the right of access, and the actual availability of the information and services necessary for its exercise. Inhibiting factors include conservative cultural traditions and national demographic interests.

From the European perspective, where government departments have taken on the major role economically and/or administratively of providing planned parenthood facilities, the role of PPAs as voluntary associations (and by extension the IPPF as a federation of these associations) is clear.

In political-philosophical terms, these bodies are vehicles for the expression of peoples' needs. While respecting the duties and responsibilities of states, they will act, where necessary, as 'counter-weights' to state authority, in defence of specific human rights. Democratic states will respect and encourage this function of voluntary associations for the sake of the common good.

In contrast to global population increase, this Regional project is undertaken against a background of increasing preoccupation by many European states with the long-term consequences of persistent low fertility, and its effect, for example, on economic growth. With governments now seriously considering means to raise fertility, it is necessary to pose the question whether they will remain sensitive to democratic values. It is for PPAs and the IPPF to act wherever individual planned parenthood rights are compromised in governments' pursuit of society's 'interests'.

Where individual rights conflict with 'social responsibilities', the Working Group on this project endorses relevant sections of the IPPF Working Group Report to the Members' Assembly and Central Council: <u>The Human Right to Family Planning</u>, 1984; in particular, paragraph 18:

> IPPF should press upon governments the realisation that only after they have demonstrated a genuine concern for the living conditions of individuals and after they have provided universal access to fertility regulation information and services will they be entitled to ask their citizens to adhere to specific population policies.

This project is an initiative of contributing PPAs, under the auspices of the IPPF Europe Region, to enhance this working relationship with the objective of maximising individual planned parenthood human rights.

Specifically, the project represents a mutual learning exercise for participating PPAs, which are able to examine planned parenthood legislation in selected countries, <u>and</u> the economic, administrative, and professional infra-structures which respective state authorities govern or indirectly control. Thus, the project's findings are primarily aimed at governments in the hope of stimulating action at this level.

It has long been recognised that social action for legal reform in this field has been a central strategy by which PPAs have fulfilled their purpose. Indeed, it has been through appeals to the fairness or unfairness of existing planned parenthood laws that PPAs and other pressure groups have enlisted the help of the state legislature against conservative social forces. However, it is well recognised that the creation of 'just' laws will not alone guarantee that means will be forthcoming. This is particularly the case with 'enabling' laws whose sole purpose is to facilitate the establishment of specific services.

Laws and Human Rights

Basic or natural rights are not always or necessarily reflected in law. However, this project recognises that planned parenthood rights may be legally ratified through their inclusion in national constitutions, bills of rights, international human rights declarations etc. The Working Group distances itself from movements opposed to its definition of planned parenthood rights which resort to idealistic philosophies (or theologies) of 'absolute rights'. Rather, a rationalist approach is adopted which recognises that all so-called 'rights' are ultimately contingent on historical conditions, and even on deterministic forces (such as medical technology) which can 'create' the conditions for certain rights literally to come into existence.

It is ultimately to an emerging global ethical consensus, enshrined in international declarations, that the Working Group refers when discussing inalienable rights contained in national legislation. While recognising that this consensus is far from total, the Group has no intention to enter theological debate on what can or cannot be a 'human right'(3), conceding that it adheres to explicit values in its position.

Restrictive and 'Enabling' Planned Parenthood Law

In the Division of Labour in Society (1893), Durkheim noted that, 'Every written law has a double object: to prescribe certain obligations and to define the sanctions which are attached to them'. The twentieth century in Europe has witnessed a swing away from injunctions against the individual making use of contraception or abortion. These injunctions stemmed from a respect for the 'natural order' of things, or, as occurred in Germany and France, out of government commitment to expansion of population. The swing began in the Soviet Union in its revolutionary period, and developed in other European countries through their own feminist struggles. Injunctions have been replaced by 'enabling' legislation which respects the right of the individual to control fertility.

It is a premise of this project that legal protection of the right to planned parenthood is ultimately desirable to ensure that family planning programmes are not adversely affected by changes of government, ideology, or threats to state-funded services.

For, although the removal of repressive legislation on planned parenthood has reduced the amount of state interference in personal affairs, the evolution of organised planned parenthood services has had the effect of binding the individual to the state in new ways.

Repressive legislation relied upon obligations directed at the individual not to practise planned parenthood on pain of punishment. The legitimisation of planned parenthood has, on the whole, shifted obligations from the individual to the state itself through its involvement in the delivery of health care in general or in its control of medical, manufacturing and consumer service standards. This is as much a bureaucratic as an economic responsibility but it is nevertheless widespread in most countries. As a result of the necessary delegation of responsibility for public services (which includes planned parenthood) from national to local government administrations, the PPA task of monitoring the quality and quantity of such services, let alone influencing any change, is now more difficult.

In sum, most European states have implicated themselves, or have been implicated, in the provision of planned parenthood, among other health and educational services, whether the 'right' to such services is legally sanctioned or not. And it is an implicit assumption of this Working Group that such involvement is inevitable, necessary and beneficial. Unfortunately, as government departments have responsibilties to many competing services within the same sphere (economically or administratively), improvements in the quality of specific services are harder to achieve.

Moreover, it is ironic that many PPAs and feminist movements have, during this century, struggled to 'nationalise' planned parenthood services - to have the government take responsibility for subsidised family planning. The bureaucratic consequences of this desired shift from the private or voluntary to the public sector are now regretted according to some feminist thinking(4).

This change of attitude merits some consideration. It should be remembered that the state has become involved in planned parenthood through the demands made upon medical services to deliver the 'technology' of certain contraceptives, abortion, sterilisation, infertility treatments etc. However, changes in contraceptive methods could eliminate the necessity for large-scale medical intervention at least in the area of contraception. This raises the question whether - at least in some areas - the right to planned parenthood could be furthered by a <u>change</u> in state health care involvement through an <u>increase</u> in individual control over methods. This possibility now has the support of the IPPF in its policy on community family planning services, something which is echoed in the statement of the 1983 IPPF Working Group report:

> Governments should take steps to facilitate the
> involvement of trained lay personnel in the delivery
> of fertility regulation services. (op. cit.paragraph
> 45)

Conclusion

Planned parenthood legislation, which PPAs have played
a vital role in creating, has subsequently complicated
their task of defending and furthering individual rights
and needs, because, for reasons described above, the free
exercise of planned parenthood legal rights must now be
measured according to the resources devoted by the state
(through medical bureaucracies, manufacturers, etc) to one
sector of health-care in competition with other sectors.
Thus in campaigning for better services PPAs themselves are
inevitably drawn into a cost-benefit evaluation of the
level of resources which the state ought to be devoting to
planned parenthood vis-à-vis other health care demands.
However, this is not to say that the project
participants propose to hold their respective governments
responsible in toto for what PPAs choose to define as
adequate practical support for planned parenthood. This
would be unreasonable in view of the criteria chosen to
define it, which arguably extend beyond the scope of
government control (for example, the availability of family
planning literature). Rather, the aim is for participants
to bring to the attention of governments and non-
governmental organisations (NGOs) examples of the failure
of certain laws, and/or conditions which they govern, to
accord with the general spirit of planned parenthood rights
as internationally understood. The Working Group hopes
that the project will provide a European yardstick or
measure to be adopted by national PPAs in their campaigning
activities.

NOTES

1. Simons, J Fertility Control in Europe, European
Population Conference 1982, EPC(82) 3-E Strasbourg.
2. See Chapter Four.
3. In contrast with the concept of planned parenthood
presented here, which among other things includes the right

to abortion, a national referendum in Ireland in 1983 resulted in accession to the foetus the right to life <u>as a basic human right</u> over and above that of a woman to decide if she is willing/able to bring a pregnancy to term. This is <u>not</u> to say that abortion is thereby an acceptable method of family planning.

4.   The so-called 'health movements' in several Western European countries constitute attempts by feminists to contest the essentially male-dominated, bureaucratic control of health care. It is argued that the right of women over their own bodies is often denied in the alienating 'medicalisation' and 'hospitalisation' of the non-illness processes of childbirth and contraception.

Chapter Two

METHODOLOGY

Evolution of the Regional Project

The Regional Project, originally entitled 'Planned Parenthood as a Basic Human Right', developed as a collaborative effort of individuals who contributed ideas and objective data at different stages in its progress between 1980 and 1984. Due to successive refinements not anticipated in the project's original formulation, it is worth briefly tracing its evolution as a Regional activity.

The First Stage (1980-1982)

At the ninth meeting of the IPPF Europe Regional Council held in Oslo in May 1980, the representatives of the Family Planning Council of Yugoslavia (FPCY), Nevenka Petric and Ziva Beltram, proposed a project to inquire into:

> the status of planned parenthood as an integral part of human rights, and into the conditions for the implementation of these human rights, on the basis of IPPF, United Nations, and other declarations on this subject. . . to survey the present situation, conditions and obstacles relating to the fulfilment of this human right, and, on the basis of the findings to elaborate a common action at the IPPF Regional level.

The FPCY had a strong historical investment in this subject (discussed further in the Sjövall paper, page 19 below) dating back to the 1950s, at which time the Federation of Women's Societies of Yugoslavia declined membership of the IPPF until the basic human right to planned parenthood was constitutionally elevated to primary position. The FPCY regards this project as a retrospective review of progress made, in IPPF Europe member countries, in realising both planned parenthood human rights (as internationally understood) both in theory and practice.

The project involved an analysis of United Nations, international and other non-governmental statements/ declarations designating planned parenthood as a human right, and an attempt to identify the degree of government commitment to these declarations in the form of national laws and services.

It was agreed that, at its broadest, the project <u>aimed to heighten peoples' consciousness of their human rights and responsibilities in planned parenthood matters</u>. Part of this task, at the Regional level, is to help reinforce the working relationship between PPAs and their national government departments responsible for planned parenthood services.

This can be done by examining legislation and the corresponding quality and extent of those planned parenthood services under government control, transnationally.

It was felt that involvement by the IPPF, as a nongovernmental organisation, would add weight to the case presented by PPAs to their governments for changes in planned parenthood law and/or services where necessary.

The 'common action' referred to recommendations which PPAs would propose to their governments in order to help overcome practical obstacles which undermine legal rights.

The first Regional Working Group meeting (convened by Freddy Deven, Belgium) identified the political-philosophical dimensions of the project, and developed a methodology for a case-study analysis of selected countries.

The scale of the task of dealing with 18 countries demanded that data collection be broken down into two forms:

- the <u>first</u> would comprise a <u>brief</u> overview of the <u>de jure/de facto</u> situations of all 18 countries, which would not go into the detail of the obstacles, etc.

- the <u>second</u> would comprise case studies of a number of selected countries, whose PPA representatives were prepared to undertake the analyses necessary to provide a comprehensive national picture of consumer utilisation of legally recognised planned parenthood services.

The Second Stage (1982-1983)

In May 1983, the second meeting of the Regional Working Group agreed on 9 issues which would be taken by IPPF Europe to encapsulate planned parenthood human rights. It is recognised that some issues are of a higher order of importance than others, and the list does not constitute an order of priority:

1   Government recognition of the human right to determine the number and spacing of children. Protection of family and child.
2   Family planning facilities and services.
3   The sale, distribution and advertisement of contraceptives.
4   Availability/sale of family planning-related literature.
5   Sterilisation.
6   Abortion.
7   Infertility treatment.
8   Sex education/family life education.
9   Adoption.

National profiles

The National Profiles (NP) comprise 18 country summaries of the de jure, and related de facto situations covering the 9 issues above according to the following criteria:

- national recognition of each issue in law - whether this legal recognition is: enabling/protective/ neutral (unlegislated)/ restrictive-repressive.
- the existence of services/facilities to which these laws relate. The involvement of government, vis-à-vis the non-governmental sector in the provision of these services/facilities.

Country Case Studies

The de jure/de facto comparison contained in the national profiles (pages 61ff) is sufficient to identify in what ways the state and/or non-governmental organisations have become involved in planned parenthood. The form which this involvement has taken is used for the purposes of the project as a measure of the 'political will' of governments to respect the spirit of international declarations on human rights.

However, the country case studies undertaken by Belgium, France, Poland, UK and Yugoslavia are intended to fulfill the project's objectives to 'survey the <u>obstacles</u> relating to the human right to planned parenthood'. While national profiles are sufficient to display <u>where</u> the difficulties and inadequacies in services, literature, education etc appear to lie, they cannot explain <u>why</u> the differences in the <u>de jure</u> and <u>de facto</u> siutations persist. Each country case study comprises:

-        an historical and political review of events leading up to the formulation of planned parenthood laws and the practical circumstances to which they relate;
-        a focus on the major gaps which persist across the nine issues;
-        an evaluation of the obstacles which are believed to prevent the free and responsible exercise of planned parenthood rights;
-        PPA recommendations to governments and other public authorities toward resolution of problems.

The Final Stage (1984)

In December 1984, the IPPF Europe Region convened a seminar in Dubrovnik, Yugoslavia to discuss the objectives and findings of the project with participants from selected PPAs and respective relevant government departments*. The latter were invited to explain the means at the disposal of, and limitations on, their governments to respond to the PPA recommendations contained in the case studies. Some aspects of the interchange between PPA and government participants are presented in the Conclusion, as a postscript to the evidence presented below.

---

*Government participants came from: France, Italy, Portugal, Spain, United Kingdom and Yugoslavia, PPA participants from: Belgium, France, Italy, Poland, Portugal, United Kingdom and Yugoslavia (see Appendix 2).

Chapter Three

THEORETICAL AND POLITICAL BACKGROUND

The Terminology of Planned Parenthood
M Kozakiewicz

The aim of this paper is to demonstrate the variety of meanings which may be attributed to the terms 'family planning', 'population policy' etc. It is easily possible to illustrate the fact that both pro- and antinatalist population policies can violate human rights. European history is replete with examples of moral and ideological justifications which have been advanced to subordinate individual control over fertility, by available means, to the population aims and needs of the state.

The manner of implementation of policies is the critical factor; in this respect, family planning can be viewed both as an aim and as a tool. One of the tasks facing the Working Group in this project is to identify the limits of planned parenthood as an individual private affair as distinct from an area of social responsibility.

It is important to note that whereas the term 'planned parenthood' is prefered to 'family planning' for the title of this project, it was nevertheless felt that the former was still unsatisfactory, for it failed to convey the notion of responsible parenthood extending over a period of time. It was agreed that 'conscious parenthood' comes closer to what the Working Group understands by 'planned parenthood'.

The original feminist movement for <u>birth control</u> was founded upon the quest for better maternal and child health, and basic sexual freedom, through access to and unfettered use of existing methods of fertility regulation. The internationalisation of the movement, and attempts at the national level to enlist the support of the public, professions and governments, led to a shift in the title to <u>family planning</u>. Apart from the greater appeal which the inclusion of the term 'family' into anything guarantees, the terminological shift also placed greater emphasis upon the objective of child-spacing through contraceptive use, rather than simply child 'prevention'. It was also felt at that time (1930s) that the movement ought to divest itself of the eugenicism which had been assumed by the pioneers a decade earlier, due to the racist and anti-working class connotations the latter increasingly evoked.

By the time the IPPF was established in 1952, the term planned parenthood was officially adopted in place of family planning to designate - in the spirit of human rights and responsibilities - that issues of reproduction are issues of social and sexual existence whose implications go beyond the structuring of the traditional family. These issues are reflected in the categories, designated by this Working Group, collectively to define planned parenthood (see page 11).

Addressing the nine issues listed here as constituting 'planned parenthood human rights', for the purpose of investigating the record of European states in the field, is somewhat of a terminological compromise itself. For certain issues have quite different historical and cultural significance for participating nations and this must be recognised in any comparative analysis of national performance. The most important example is sterilisation, which for certain countries has no legal and/or functional status as a routine method of 'contraception'.

Another terminological compromise, within the historical development of the IPPF, implicitly matched population reduction with the 'health-promoting endeavour' of family planning/planned parenthood as a human right. However, in counterposing the notion of population control as commonly understood, against that of planned parenthood in human rights terms, it is necessary - in the European context - to rescue the term population policy from this dichotomy. It is argued that there is no necessary contradiction between a national population policy per se and respect for planned parenthood human rights.

Although the term population policy evokes, at face value, the notion of a combined political-economic and social strategy consciously adopted by a government to achieve a desired demographic objective, in real terms it has no such simple objective meaning. For it may also be used analytically to define a collection of relatively uncoordinated social (rather than strictly demographic-related) policies pursued by government for unrelated ends, which may, however, have demographic consequences. That is, they can have a latent causal effect on fertility behaviour.

- 14 -

Population policies may be 'consciously' formulated to achieve three demographic objectives - described by the terms 'antinatalist', 'pronatalist' and 'neutral'.

Antinatalist population policies incorporate strategies of birth limitation for macro-economic ends. Here contraceptive methods and services are employed through a variety of legal and administrative measures to restrict child bearing - in order to 'adjust' the pace of socio-economic development. It is possible to identify non-repressive antinatalistic policies which seek to achieve such ends through mass education and various incentives. However, examples exist in developing countries where contraception has been strategically deployed to actually limit individual free-choice concerning family size, thus violating the principle of planned parenthood as a basic human right.

In contrast, **pronatalist** population policies may be employed where low fertility is believed to pose a threat to the socio-economic standards a national population enjoys. In the absence of population replacement from other sources (eg. immigration) 'excessive' fertility decline disrupts the education system initially, and subsequently affects the labour supply, the contribution of the economically active sector to social welfare, etc.

The histories of developed European countries with characteristically low birth rates have seen the imposition of repressive pronatalist policies for a variety of chauvinist, imperialist and racist reasons. These have taken the form of legal injunctions against contraceptive practice. Moral and economic pressures can also be used in order to compel women/couples to have more children.

However, pronatalist population policies developed in recent times, particularly in most Eastern European states, have sought, in most cases, not to restrict the freedom of individuals to decide on the number and spacing of their children (through control of fertility regulation supplies or services) - at least overtly(1) - but to eliminate obstacles to childbearing through a variety of financial and other incentives to potential parents.

A final category of **neutral** policy on population should also be noted in those countries where the official view is that the prevailing population trend cannot easily be manipulated for economic ends. In addition, a state declaring a 'neutral' policy may, indeed, secretly wish to influence population for economic or other ends, but desists for ideological reasons. For example, such activity might threaten the national popularity of the government, or stand in the face of an espoused liberalism.

The absence of any demonstrable population-related policies or demographic concerns should not conceal the fact that a number of socio-economic policies, which combine to influence individual decisions regarding family size, can operate, de facto, in anti- or pronatalist ways. The case of the United Kingdom is pertinent here, where there is official 'neutrality' on the subject of population. As Eversley has noted, in the face of the consequences of 'natural' demographic fluctuations the current general socio-economic policies of government have an antinatalist effect upon couples. Consequently, changes in a range of socio-economic measures would be required to negate this effect. Previous family-related economic policies acted to place the competitive situation of the traditional two-child family (concerning purchase of living space, consumer goods, etc) on par with childless couples. This was achieved through variable taxation and the allocation of benefits. However:

. . . limitations on public spending which began in the mid-1970s. . . mean that the system has now become a punitive one, and that families with children can compete, year on year, ever less successfully with the all-earner households. The immediate response to the fall in the number of births was to cut teacher education and to reduce capital and current expenditure on education, health and housing probably faster than the fall in births would justify. . . so that the equality of delivery services and the possibility of access to them, declined. The question is whether or not this does in fact constitute, implicitly or explicitly, intentionally or unintentionally, a population policy. If we introduce or perpetuate a system which, whatever its original intentions, comes to penalise parents, in their own estimation, for reproducing at all, or for having two children rather than one, or three rather than two, the motivation for birth control becomes very strong indeed. One might call it the policy of disendowment, and it is disingenuous to believe that it will not have a negative effect on reproduction (2).

De facto population policy may always be identified as operating as consequences of societies' economic and social welfare planning. To this extent, the human right to planned parenthood will also always be modulated by social organisation. However, while a population policy can never be 'neutral' in respect of the practice of planned parenthood, such a policy does not have to have a discernably <u>negative</u> effect on free choice in this field.

Conversely, human rights can be compromised through pronatalist, antinatalist and so-called 'neutral' population policies. For it is not the type of population policy but the way in which it is implemented (the precise nature and effect of incentives/disincentives) which decides whether planned parenthood human rights can be regarded as violated or not.

In conclusion the following examples of China and Romania have both provided illustrations of unacceptable uses of population policies.

The **Chinese** concept of family planning is an example of subordination of this right to the socio-economic needs of the state. This was apparent in the 1950s when an openly pronatalist policy was advocated and promoted: 'The larger the population, the more numerous the hands, and therefore, the greater the total production'.(3) The same situation pertains in the 1980s, where an equally energetic antinatalist policy is promoted by means of unequivocal endorsement of fertility control through a 'one child per couple' drive throughout the nation.

In an 'Open letter on population control' of the 25th August 1980, issued by the Central Committee of the Communist Party of China, it was stated: 'If a population increases too fast, the accumulation of funds will decrease. If the population increases slowly, the accumulation of funds will increase. Now please think it over. What a great positive role the money saved from this will play when it is used to develop the economy, culture and education'.(4) This is an almost classical formulation of the Malthusian thesis. The incompatibility of such a concept of family planning with human rights lies not so much in the formulation of antinatalist goals but in the ways and means used to achieve them: psychological, political, financial and moral pressures; criminalisation of those having second pregnancies etc.

A study by I Ceterchi et al of the situation in **Romania** concludes that, 'Family planning within the meaning of Romanian law is founded on full respect for the human right of every family to decide on the number and spacing of their children'. Nevertheless, the Romanian government places strong limitations on the individual's freedom to control fertility. This is justified by means of an ideological stance based on the premise that family planning is an inextricable part of socio-economic planning for which all individuals are responsible. National economic development is therefore interpreted to mean: 'Each family should endeavour to have at least four children, so that the next generation should be numerically superior to the present one'.(5)

Of contraceptives: only 'natural methods' are declared to be in their nature outside legal preoccupations. Of other methods only condoms are permitted (if they can be obtained). The remaining methods may be legally used by those women who fulfil those criteria necessary to obtain a legal abortion, viz:

- the life of the mother would be at risk from a pregnancy;
- eugenic reasons/threat of serious malformation;
- pregnancy resulting from rape;
- the woman is over 40 years old and therefore may imperil the physical and psychological condition of the child;
- the woman has already given birth to four children, which she must provide for alone.

Both aborter and abortee are penalised when these conditions are not fulfilled. Moreover, the mere possession of any special instruments or any other means for the interruption of pregnancy outside of special health institutions, is also punishable.

Planned Parenthood in the Context of Human Rights
T Sjövall

Introduction

What follows are some rather sketchy reflections on the development of the ideological climate, particularly in the Western world, during this century and its implications for a planned parenthood movement with ever-increasing ambitions for global applicability and impetus. The ideas expressed are to an extent drawn from a paper presented at the IPPF Anniversary Conference at Brighton in 1973 under the title "Planned Parenthood Reconsidered: Human Rights and Welfare Aspects". The various organised activities undertaken in our field, nationally as well as internationally, are referred to as the 'Movement'. Special attention is given to current phrases designating the Movement because of the unspoken associations they may evoke and the presumed influence such associations might have on attitudes towards human rights.

Ideological Developments

Birth Control

It is interesting to note in this context that an organised Movement began with a clear but restricted ambition to promote what were regarded as human rights at the end of the last century and the first decades of the present one. The pioneers were mostly women engaged in the emerging struggle for improved general life conditions of contemporary womanhood and particularly impressed by the misery they met among fellow sisters as a consequence of unwanted pregnancy and/or children. The phrase chosen for their activities was 'birth control', and it was regarded as a more or less exclusive female concern.

The concrete manifestations of the Movement occurred in the form of birth control services for women established in some European countries and the USA. The methods available at the time were only so-called barrier ones, and sterilisation under special conditions in a few countries.

Aletta Jacobs founded a clinic in Amsterdam in 1881. Marie Stopes' Mothers' Clinic for Constructive Birth Control was founded in London in 1921, and Margaret Sanger opened a birth control clinic in New York in 1923(6).

It is worth recalling too, that in 1920 the Soviet Government legalised abortion on request, to alleviate the detrimental effects of illegal abortion on women's health, though a restrictive law was introduced in 1936 and abortion law was again liberalised only in 1955.

In order to spread the message, an international conference on the subject was held in Zurich in 1930, with the special aim of reaching and enlisting the support of the medical profession with the indispensable 'scientific' respectability it could bring to the subject. This aim was to some extent achieved at the Zurich meeting, but in an attempt to avoid the somewhat technical connotation adhering to the term 'birth control' it was around that time that this was exchanged for the term 'family planning'. The importance of words should not be underestimated, and this particular change obviously widened the scope of the Movement to include men as well as children, at least in principle.

Family Planning

During World War II the initiative taken at Zurich for international cooperation in our field was of course almost entirely interrupted. However, family planning activities continued nationally in various countries under very diverse conditions, ensuring that the Movement was here to stay.

The war catastrophe, including the first appearance on the scene of weapons of mass human destruction, had profoundly changed the entire predicament of mankind even if the implications of this do not seem to have been clearly realised until very recently. The predominant ideological climate after World War II was that this will not and must not happen again if we only take reasonable precautions on the basis of our experiences and our proliferating scientific development. No doubt the war also brought a changed perspective on population problems in that several countries, under the influence of heavy human losses during the war, adopted a pronatalist policy.

For the first time an explicit national political dimension was added to controversies between pronatalist and fertility restrictive ideologies, so far dominated by socio-cultural and religious arguments.

On a global scale this politicisation of the subject was reflected, during some 30 years after the war, in a division of the world into two blocs regarding preferred fertility-restrictive methods. In the Eastern part of Europe widespread induced abortion was practised, almost to the exclusion of other methods, whereas in the Western part contraceptive methods were preferred with a gradual legalislation of induced abortion as a reasonable complement in cases where contraception had failed. Such a division in political blocs is obviously not promotive of 'universal human rights'. It represented of course a very large-scale trend only, and differences in countries in all parts of the world were, and still are, very considerable. However, viewed globally this division on a political basis was certainly very conspicuous at the time.

By far the most important consequence of the war in our context was, however, the establishment of the United Nations. This aimed at promoting global interaction and legislation on a global basis, with particular emphasis on ethical and human rights aspects as expressed at a number of world conferences and in declarations during the years to follow. The UN Declaration of Human Rights of 1948 avowed, among other things, freedom of thought, speech and the dissemination of information and knowledge through all available channels, as well as the right to education and to participation in scientific achievements and advantages for all individuals. Of great importance for our Movement, in close cooperation with the medical profession, was also the broad definition of health given in the Constitution of the World Health Organisation of the same year, namely as 'a state of complete physical, mental and social well-being, and not merely the absence of disease and infirmity'.

General well-being was proclaimed as a basic human right, and if taken seriously, in spite of being somewhat utopian, continues to have considerable implications for our Movement in its capacity as a health-promoting organisation.

In 1946, prior to these UN declarations Elise Ottesen-Jensen of Sweden had convened an international conference in Stockholm in order to follow up the initiatives taken in Zurich in 1930. At this Stockholm meeting the overall aim for future activities was formulated as follows: 'To promote the physical and spiritual health, welfare and happiness of the individual, the family and society in a new and united world'. Among the resolutions adopted in support of this aim the very first one stated: 'Every child has a right to be wanted by both parents, and all parents have the right to decide upon the number of children they shall bring to the world'. The other resolutions emphasised 'scientific' aspects of our field, presumably in a continued appeal to the medical profession.

The general atmosphere of this meeting could well be said to have been dominated by the issue of human rights as a basic principle. Particularly noteworthy in this respect was the explicit reference to the rights of the child, a crucial human rights aspect which since then has been practically lost in the general debate until recently.

The pioneers of the Movement at this time, including Elise Ottesen-Jensen and myself, were no doubt impressed by the contemporary so-called neo-Malthusians in believing that after World War II, which must never be repeated, the most threatening concrete global problem was that of 'overpopulation'. In addition, we were influenced by our ambition to collect and engage as many groups and organisations as possible with interests related to our own.

The next international conference in our field, following up the Stockholm meeting, took place at Cheltenham in 1948 under the title 'Population and World Resources'. Here several participants with a strong neo-Malthusian inclination spoke, and the overall spirit of the conference, as reflected in the resolutions, was that family planning is more or less synonymous with the application of contraceptive techniques, and this should be regarded as essentially instrumental for global population control.

Again, the family planning pioneers did not sufficiently realise at the time the implications of this development in terms of an ideological division between individual human rights proponents of family planning on the one side, and 'scientific' and political ones of population control on the other.

Nevertheless, in connection with the Cheltenham conference and the period leading to the foundation of the

IPPF in 1952 the descriptive concept of 'family planning' for our Movement was, so to speak, officially substituted by 'planned parenthood' although this has hardly been systematically reflected in everyday language, even today. The concept of 'planned parenthood' designated in the name of the Federation may nevertheless be seen as reflecting a realistic consideration of the fact that problems connected with reproduction and parenthood to an ever increasing extent go far beyond the realm of the traditional family. Informed, conscious or planned parenthood, taken seriously, includes all human rights aspects in our field, from appropriate information about 'facts of life' in early childhood and onwards to the individual human right to knowledge and means for restricting or promoting fertility at reproductive age. For those adhering to a basic human rights attitude it therefore seems essential to adopt consequently and consistently the term 'planned parenthood' for an overall designation of our activities in the field.

Planned Parenthood

When the first Constitution of the IPPF was adopted at a meeting in Stockholm in 1953, the statement: 'the belief that a favourable balance between the populations and natural resources of the world is an indispensable condition of a lasting world peace' was put as a first paragraph of that document. No doubt this constituted a sort of legitimation, particularly for the US member organisation supported by the British, to present IPPF policy in speeches and publications during the following decade from a rather lopsided population control angle at the expense of the original emphasis on human rights aspects. This trend was accentuated by the fact that the international secretariat was located in London and that our official language was and is English. An ideological division in these respects within the Federation between the US and Britain on one side and the rest of the former Europe, Near East and African Region (ENEA) on the other side started to make its appearance.

In the latter part of the '50s, this was substantiated in a concrete and thought-provoking way when in our continual efforts to recruit more member organisations, we were told by the Federation of Women's Societies of Yugoslavia, nationally active in our field, that having studied available IPPF printed material where 'the

Malthusian theory is taken into consideration as being the basic method for achieving social progress', they could not envisage membership 'for the time being'. The implication was that this women's organisation could only subscribe to a more explicit emphasis on human rights in accord with the spontaneous and self-evident attitude of the first pioneer women in other parts of the West. This should, of course, be regarded as an important historical background to the fact that it was the present Yugoslav member association which took the initiative in Europe to organise the Regional Working Group on Planned Parenthood as a Basic Human Right, here presenting its final report.

Partly as a result of this declaration of the Yugoslav Federation of Women's Societies, the Regional Executive Committee decided to press for a change in the wording of the controversial section of the IPPF Constitution in the sense of placing planned parenthood as a fundamental human right first, explicitly emphasising the interest of family welfare, and to include psychological aspects in training and education in various fields to promote our aims.

These changes to the Constitution, adopted at the IPPF Governing Body meeting in Singapore 1963, contributed to a considerable increase of member associations of the ENEA Region in the following years.

In an overall perspective the 1960s are frequently referred to as the decade of youth revolution in the West, bringing to the fore various manifestations of youth protest in many countries against being insufficiently involved and respected in a period of rapid cultural development. One could also speak of an explicit demonstration of ideological conflict between the generations, illustrating a special dimension of the human rights issue, namely the fact of mutual interdependence as well as the need for a more systematic cooperation between individuals and groups of individuals. This contributed to initiatives within the IPPF during the following years to define certain "groups at risk", including adolescents, in terms of the promotion of human rights.

In 1965, the first government financial support of the IPPF was granted by Sweden, followed in 1967 by the USA. The emphasis from these financial sources was definitely on providing modern contraceptive techniques and services to "developing countries" in the conviction that this would be the most appropriate way of curbing the "population bomb" or the world "population explosion".

This idea was of course most attractive to contraceptive manufacturers, and introduced a considerable ingredient of financial interest within the planned parenthood movement. The idea as such, however, completely disregarded the fact that a reasonable balance of population had been achieved in the Northern hemisphere without any extensive practise of instrumental contraception, a fact that began to be more seriously considered in the late 1960s.

These circumstances influenced the ideological climate at the time in a political and commercial rather than in a human rights direction. Meanwhile, however, several bodies within the UN started to pay increasing attention to planned parenthood, with a clear emphasis on human rights aspects. The most important expression of this was an extension of the Declaration of Human Rights of 1948, made at the 20th Anniversary Conference in Teheran in 1968, to the effect that 'couples have a basic human right to decide freely and responsibly on the number and spacing of their children and a right to adequate education and information in this respect'.

The 1970s were marked by a number of international conferences and conventions organised by the UN as well as by the various nongovernmental organisations with interests related to planned parenthood. To an increasing extent representatives from developing countries achieved full membership at these international events which contributed to a strong emphasis on human rights as leading principles for global development.

The UN Population Conference, held in Bucharest in 1974, may be regarded as a breakthrough, revealing that the prevailing efforts at the indiscriminate and isolated introduction of various 'developed' country technologies, including fertility regulation, in developing countries were unsuccessful at all levels. Every development effort has to be subject to careful planning, with due consideration being given to the individual as well as the local socio-cultural environment.

'Integration' became a slogan of the decade for efforts and activities aimed at achieving national and international progress and development. Other such slogans were 'primary health care' and 'community based distribution' of information and services everywhere.

The Bucharest Conference also led to a bridging of the gap between the two aforementioned global blocs with regard to preferred techniques of fertility regulation, resulting in an increased acceptance of contraceptive methods in Eastern Europe and a gradual legalisation of induced abortion elsewhere in Europe.

All these circumstances paved the way, at least in theory, towards free choice on the part of the individual in matters of planned parenthood, presumably based on 'informed consent' in regard of the preferred technical method, including abortion and sterilisation.

In a special IPPF position paper published as a response to the Bucharest Conference the ideological foundation of the Movement on basic human rights was strongly and persistently emphasised and this was also the case in IPPF official declarations and proclamations during the years to follow. It is noteworthy, though, that in all these documents the phrase 'family planning' has regularly been chosen to designate our activities, in spite of the official name given to the Federation.

In 1977, IPPF undertook a self-assessment of its role, objectives and activities with a view to establishing directions for its future work. The study, which was conducted in consultation with all member associations, showed conclusively that 'The IPPF's major and primary policy - to promote family planning as a basic human right . . . is to remain the number one flag of the Federation as whole'. It was also recognised that there was a need for renewed and more concerted efforts to turn this policy objective into reality.

Promotion of family planning as a basic human right was identified as one of the priority areas for action in the IPPF's 1982-84 and 1985-87 Plans. To facilitate the implementation of this policy a Working Group was established in 1982 to examine the major issues involved in the exercise of the right to family planning and to make recommendations for its more vigorous promotion. The report of the Group constituted one of the most substantive discussion topics at the IPPF's Third Members' Assembly in November 1983, accentuating the Federation's renewed focus on this major area of its work.

Some general reflections

The so-called developed countries of Europe and North America have until recently regarded themselves as self-evidently more knowledgable and sophisticated than other cultures of the world, mainly on the basis of their achievements in technology and natural sciences, even to the extent of equating illiteracy with stupidity. In this respect a remarkable change has occurred in the ideological climate of their thinking in recent years, in that the so-called humanistic sciences such as anthropology, sociology and human psychology, although not translatable into the conceptual framework of the natural sciences, are becoming recognised as an indispensable complement to these natural sciences in our efforts to understand 'human nature'. Here the word 'integration' as applied to different fields of human experience and knowledge achieves its true significance.

Much of the European version of human psychology, a fundamental field of knowledge for the conceptualisation of the nature and predicament of man, was, in the first decades after the Second World War, strongly influenced by the theories of Sigmund Freud and his followers. These theories described man predominately on the basis of biological equipment and propensities, thereby remaining within the respected realm of natural sciences but at a certain expense of psycho-social and cultural influences. In this view there was a tendency to regard man as a complicated technical structure or apparatus that in due time would be exhaustively explained and understood in chemical and physical terms.

Human sciences on the other hand are concerned with human behaviour, including individual mental functioning, and particularly with human interactions and relationships. What has generally been recognised more recently is the fundamental importance of such relationships, independent of individual biological equipment, for the development of 'human nature'. We now realise that no individual can be adequately understood, nor can his behaviour be relatively predicted, without careful consideration of his interpersonal, social and cultural environment. In this ideological perspective what has been particularly emphasised is the importance of values and value-systems for the formation of man; that is, precisely those phenomena which cannot be adequately described or understood within the theoretical framework of the natural sciences. It is obviously within this context that the promotion of human rights finds its proper place.

It is of course not easy to define exactly which human values and evaluations, on which human rights are based, could and should be regarded as truly 'universal' or 'basic'. In the absence of a catalogue derived from anthropological study we can only guess. In so doing we may assume that a basic urge for the preservation of life is a reasonable foundation for the evaluation of individual survival as a universal human right.

However, contemporary human psychology has demonstrated that 'survival' has a different 'existential' meaning in poor and rich areas of the world. In the former it is essentially a question of physical survival: 'as long as there is life there is hope'. In the rich areas, on the other hand, with their highly developed material welfare systems 'survival' has acquired a more symbolic connotation in terms of the individual experience of having an identity, the essential manifestation of which is a reasonably steadfast and functioning personal value system. A predominant mental 'symptom' in contemporary welfare society is hopelessness in regard to an immediate subjective experience of 'being somebody': 'as long as there is hope there is life'. Lack of such identity-feeling proves in clinical experience to be emotionally equivalent to a threat to physical survival and should, accordingly, be taken very seriously.

Now parenthood happens to have a very profound significance for both those aspects of human survival, because 'my' child, being half made up from my very bodily substance and, granted the probability of him/her surviving me, represents the most obvious and concrete manifestation of my own physical survival. On the other hand, my child, being reared and fostered in accordance with my personal value system, represents symbolically the survival of my identity. Both these aspects provide for the parent a so far underestimated subjective experience of continuity and meaning in life. That child-rearing means transmitting the parental value-system to children is a fact and an inevitable constituent of the family institution rather than a <u>human right</u>. Obviously it implies the danger of violating what may be regarded as the human rights of the children. However, the awareness of and the reaction to this danger has never been stronger than it is today in our part of the world.

Moreover, and somewhat paradoxically, one of the most frequent complaints met in clinical practice today is that the parents were not firm enough, were not consistent in setting limits and boundaries, and this is experienced as lovelessness from their side.

In summary, granted that survival, in various existential interpretations of that concept, may be considered a fundamental right of every human being born to this world, parenthood has a more central and concrete significance for the experiential predicament of man than anything else. Taken seriously, this illuminates the unacceptable simplicity of any one-sided contraceptive policy and even the actual violation of human rights inherent in such a policy. It also illustrates the ethical necessity of taking more than technical and biological facts into account in planned parenthood practice all over the world.

Another evaluation which may be regarded as fairly universal implies that whatever you claim to be your honest belief or conviction should be adequately reflected in your behaviour and actions. However, this particular principle seems to be severely violated nowadays, in that all solemn declarations and proclamations on human rights at the international level, even when signed by a number of states, seem to be poorly reflected in concrete actions and practice all over the world. The resulting damage to human relationships penetrates to all strata of populations and to an increasing extent marks contemporary everday behaviour in the form of widespread dishonest and violence. This is as much a threat to the physical survival of mankind as the nuclear arms race itself. It is this conviction and spirit more than anything else that motivated the investigation of this Working Group.

Defending Planned Parenthood Rights: the Role of the PPA, IPPF, and the State

P Meredith

In international meetings which have followed from the 1974 Bucharest World Population Conference (for example: the Proceedings of the Symposium on Population and Human Rights, Vienna 1981; Council of Europe European Population Conference, Strasbourg 1982), government advisers and social scientists have turned their attention toward the moral issues raised by the emergence of population policies; that is, by the rectitude of state interference in fertility behaviour in pursuit of the common good.

The purpose of this paper is to examine the problems which this development poses for planned parenthood associations, which stand as intermediaries between state and individual in the defence and promotion of fertility regulation rights. European associations collaborating in this IPPF project lay open to question their own 'proper' function in this relationship. The rationale behind the project takes into account two developments common to Europe which are believed to have far reaching implications for PPA policies and activities in the future.

The first development concerns the extent to which European states have taken control over and responsibility for the provision of fertility regulation services for their populations. Consequently, PPAs must defend planned parenthood rights not merely to the public but to governments, being the primary authority for social change. This complicates the task of defending and furthering the interests of family planning more than would be the case if PPAs, themselves, had economic and administrative control in this sphere. However, both the enormous scale of social and economic administration of national fertility regulation services, and the degree to which these services

The author would like to thank C Alison McIntosh, University of Michigan, for comments on an earlier draft of this paper.

are indivisible from broader medical health care systems, have acted to elevate government departments to primary positions of power and in most cases to marginalise the influence of voluntary associations. Within the framework of this project the PPA is obliged to decide whether planned parenthood rights are sufficiently respected in terms of resources allocated by government, in view of competing demands from other sectors for which the latter is responsible.

The second development is a continuation of low fertility rates in Europe which are increasingly perceived as harbouring negative social and economic consequences. Many governments feel a responsibility to respond to these low rates, with measures to stimulate birth-rates. PPAs should recognise that this may reduce government enthusiasm to further what are in effect individual rights to limit births through the allocation of additional resources.

The objective here is to examine conflicts of obligation confronting both PPAs and their governments as a result of these developments. The obligation to campaign for/provide the means for the full exercise of planned parenthood rights is compromised by the need to recognise/manage constraints on allocation of scarce health care resources (and the future economy in general). The final section below considers the potential conflict between parental rights versus the rights of young people to planned parenthood information and services. An examination of the division of labour between PPAs and the governments under which they function raises the question of IPPF's role in this relationship.

Rights and Responsibilities: IPPF

In Planned Parenthood in the Context of Human Rights (pages 19ff), Sjövall described how the 'globalisation' of national planned parenthood issues can influence, for good or ill, the specific functional relationship PPAs have as voluntary associations with the states within which they operate. This might be described in terms of a constructive 'tension' of specific versus general interests. IPPF, as a federation of voluntary associations, began, Sjövall reminds us, as a movement designed to further the rights of individual women on a trans-national scale. In this respect, the IPPF also complies with the function of a voluntary association as described by De Tocqueville in 1835.

> Through voluntary associations, individuals can make
> their claims audible; without them they are
> inarticulate, or a drowned confused babble of voices.
> If the state, itself, is to satisfy their diverse
> needs, free associations provide the channels through
> which its members' experiences and claims can be
> expressed. The lonely individual confronting the
> state is dwarfed and overawed; its vast impersonality
> induces a sense of hopeless frustration. By
> association he gains strength to bend state policy to
> cater more for his interests . . . (6)

Thus, in principle, the role of the IPPF, as a
federation of such associations, is also to intercede on
behalf of individuals, where necessary, against the
managerial imperatives of states. If, as is argued below,
population management is an inevitable and even necessary
responsibility of states, then IPPF's brief mirrors that of
its member associations: to monitor as part of its work the
extent to which the activities of the state - as manager of
all social 'interests' - poses a threat to the sectional
interests of planned parenthood, or responds to peoples'
planned parenthood needs.

The management of populations as **masses** with competing
demands and expectations is the raison d'être of the
state. In this respect, the interests of the state rarely,
if ever, coincide with the particular interests of all
sections or individuals within it. The state is obliged in
one way or another to manage individuals in what are
perceived as the interests of the totality. Defining the
'greater good' of the totality over any single individual
or individuals is fraught with moral compromise and can
only be achieved with the greatest degree of democratic
participation.

The mass transfer of contraceptives through the IPPF
from one nation state to another, on behalf of some Third
World countries, may be seen to implicate the IPPF in the
'management' of population. The greater the part it plays
(or is requested to play) in decisions which are related to
demographic objectives, the more it becomes allied, by
default, with the managerial imperatives of 'host' states.
Where criticism exists in a grant-receiving country of the
approaches adopted by its government to population the

issue of 'sectional' versus 'general' interests is raised. This is not to suggest that the presence of demographic policies alone is a reason to refuse IPPF aid, but that the IPPF could find itself caught between the demographic interests of governments and the needs and wishes of those groups it was founded to serve.

This project, at one level, represents a reassertion of a philosophy of individualism over one of 'populationism' - a term which describes demographic planning through the manipulation of fertility regulation rights and services. However crudely or subtley engineered, it may be argued that populationism is an inevitable part of state management of the totality(7).

Sjövall's point is that whatever the weaknesses of the feminist-inspired individualism on which the movement was founded, in practice IPPF is more in accord with the role of a non-governmental organisation, and as far as fertility regulation is concerned, carries far fewer risks for the objects of its attention than the alternative political stance.

Low Fertility and Pronatalism in Europe: the PPA position

The international reaction to perceived excessive population increase in some Third World countries contrasts with the less-publicised concern of many European governments with 'excessive' fertility decline. The introduction of laws enabling fertility regulation contributed to a decline in natural increase rates, though these were not, at face value, introduced with explicit demographic/political intentions. For example, in the Netherlands, a list of such measures would include: subsidies to family planning associations; display and sale of non-prescription contraceptives; quality control regulations; special promotion of family planning among high-risk groups; and the inclusion of provision for sterilisation in medical benefit schemes.

By the early 1970s, fertility in the West had fallen far below the level required for replacement of the population in the long term. In the face of similar trends, vigorous pronatalist measures have been introduced in Eastern European countries in an effort to increase the number of births. From the point of view of the State, low fertility and declining rates of population growth pose problems for the management of society. Changes in age-structure and the growing number of elderly increase the strain on social security systems; de-population of rural areas frustrates regional development policies.(8)

Consequently, low population growth has reached the political agenda in virtually all European nations. Convergence of demographic trends may be contrasted with different governmental reaction to them. In Eastern Europe, McIntosh has noted that 5 of the 7 low fertility countries started to implement comprehensive policies intended to encourage childbearing, though among western nations only France is seriously attempting to raise the birth-rate(9).

Birth rates fell significantly in Eastern Europe in the late 1950s when most of the Socialist countries followed the example of the Soviet Union and legalised abortion on request. The demand for abortions in Romania was regarded as contributing towards a demographic disaster, and its government reacted towards this in a way very different from other Eastern European governments. At the end of 1966, its government imposed restrictions which made legal abortion virtually impossible to obtain. It also banned the importation and local manufacture of contraceptives. As a consequence, couples quickly found other ways to avoid conception or resorted to illegal abortion.

Though it had introduced a variety of incentives to child-bearing, the German Democratic Republic nevertheless introduced a liberal abortion law in 1972. Correspondingly, in the early 1960s Bulgaria, Czechoslovakia and Hungary, attempted to eliminate obstacles to childbearing: for example, by reducing the difficulties experienced by women who have to care for young children while holding a full time job; creating kindergarten places and offering paid leave from work. In addition, steps have been taken to reduce the financial burden of children through maternity and family allowances. However, in contrast to the GDR, all three countries have also placed some restrictions on access to legal abortion, especially in the case of a first or second child - by insisting that women seeking abortion appear before a special commission to obtain permission for the operation. This procedure may be itself a potent deterrent to legal abortion. These countries have, however, attempted to make modern contraceptives more widely available. Poland has also utilised family allowances, birth grants and paid or unpaid maternity leave for pronatalist purposes.

Against this background, most European governments have nevertheless agreed that their demographic objectives and responsibilities do not, in principle, extend to interference with reproduction itself. As signatories to the Proclamation of Teheran in 1968, they affirmed the basic human right of couples to determine . . . the number . . . of children they have. Chesnais draws the following inference from this act:

> The state cannot therefore interfere with individual family plans; its task is an instrumental one, which simply entails helping couples to fulfill their wishes. In other words, its role is not to influence choices but to ensure that choices become a reality. Thus, paradoxically, state intervention does not consist of restricting freedom, but on the contrary, in enhancing it, for the state's role is to ensure that the fundamental freedom to choose how many children to have exists in practice and not just in theory.(10)

In most Western nations the recent period of fertility decline has also been one of liberal abortion reform and free availability of family planning services and supplies. The most common response to this decline has been to upgrade the level of assistance to families.

It can be concluded that there is a strong tendency in Europe, over the last 30 years, for states to make concessions to individual rights in the area of fertility regulation. As a reaction to fertility decline, with some exceptions repressive pronatalist legislation has given way to, at best, a benign pronatalism in the form of financial and other incentives to childbearing. And it is fair to say that this approach is <u>not</u> regarded by PPAs or others as infringing upon individuals' designated rights to fertility regulation.(11) On the contrary, following the introduction of more liberal legislation in this field, state involvement in the provision of fertility regulation services is accepted as an indication of national recognition of the rights of women in particular.

It is arguable, however, that this involvement should be no cause for complacency by PPAs, who may have willingly relinquished control of contraceptive services at point in their histories.

Individuals' dependence on state-funded/administered services is, in most European countries, so great that it is merely necessary for these states to under-fund, or otherwise limit (or permit the limitation of) such services, for rights to planned parenthood to be compromised or even revoked in practice.

Why should this be a cause for PPA concern at this time? In the light of the issues introduced in this paper it is proposed that the involvement of the state in the economic administration or delivery of fertility regulation services at a greater level than professional/voluntary organisations complicates its general societal managerial functions. For as controller of major financial and other resources it must weigh competing demands from all spheres of society. It is for voluntary associations or related professional groups to represent planned parenthood. Hypothetically the resulting tension between the state and these groups should be constructive rather than destructive because the former cannot itself, in view of its managerial responsibilities at the macro level, also represent the spectrum of interests at the micro level. In the past 25-30 years, PPAs have been relatively successful in enlisting the sympathy of governments in furthering women's fertility regulation rights against the interests of anti-family planning and other conservative/moral pressure groups.

However, a perception of the consequences of 'excessive' fertility decline, particularly within a climate of political conservatism, is likely to lead to greater incentives to childbearing/disincentives to childlessness. To date, most European states have resorted to rather soft measures to influence behaviour in this sphere in the face of their efforts to facilitate family limitation.

McIntosh concludes that 'while increases in allowances may be substantial, governments deny a demographic objective and claim that the purpose of the transfers is to offset the degradation of living standards experienced by families with children'.

For it is a fact that the continuation of fertility decline is an expression of the use made by individuals of their right to decide on the number of children they produce by means of the fertility regulation services placed at their disposal.(12)

This raises the possibility that states may now be unable to reverse or even stem the process of fertility decline - in view of the limitations on financial or other incentives they are able to offer without negative economic consequences elsewhere. They may be forced into the difficult position of being 'guarantors' of the resources which are necessary in order to realise fertility regulation rights, while being forced to confront the fact that 'excessive' exercise of these rights lies at the heart of their demographic-economic problems.

As manager of fertility regulation resources, the state is in a position to give planned parenthood services and education low priority without appearing to renege on its commitment to uphold planned parenthood rights. Whether or not such action (or inaction) of the state is viewed cynically as a covert expression of a desire to stimulate the birth rate, the state supervises a wide variety of mechanisms which can <u>inhibit</u> the public's free exercise of such rights. These stem from the sheer complexity of the health and social welfare administration under state direction. The control of planned parenthood services, including the education necessary to be able to use them, is of necessity delegated to the appropriate regional, bureaucratic and professional authorities. Such delegation involves a significant loss of control as each section of this administration decides according to its <u>own</u> principles and priorities the quantity and quality of services or resources to be made available.

It is well established that within most European states there are powerful forces within this kind of system (for example, medical and professional educational groups, health administrators) which for moral, political, economic or even demographic reasons attempt to substitute governmental or legal directives with their own. Leaving aside maladministration, inefficiency and inadequate funding which have no particular motive, the complexity of this power structure indicates that there is little merit, in most cases, in apportioning 'blame' to civil servants or government officials for this state of affairs.

The difficult task facing PPAs is two-fold: firstly, to provide the arguments necessary to convince the state authorities that demographic-economic problems can be overcome in the long-term without abandoning the active promotion of planned parenthood rights.

Secondly, PPAs are obliged to identify what may be

defined as 'contraventions' of planned parenthood rights and propose practical and realistic recommendations to government to correct or resist them.

It is strategically useful to enlist or retain the sympathy and support of government in this task; for it is questionable whether most PPAs can now influence service provision in total confrontation with the state. As this sympathy and support has been secured from most post-war European governments, to what extent can they reasonably expect PPA cooperation in encouraging a population to act 'responsibly' in producing less or more children so as to safeguard future economic stability?

In their respective contributions to the 1982 European Conference on Population, demographers Chesnais and Van den Brekel(13) consider this question in the context of the rights and limitations of state interference in fertility behaviour, though neither provide solutions of sufficient practical value for PPA action.

Chesnais accedes <u>non-acceptibility</u> of state intervention to <u>limit</u> the practice of fertility regulation, but adds that it is the right and duty of the state to provide incentives which influence reproductive behaviour. These, he believes, should be limited to welfare policy measures whose <u>enabling</u> effect is to secure generational replacement to protect the economic status of future members of society. However, he adds, 'any propaganda . . likely to undermine couples' freedom of choice is to be condemned'. In response to the scenario posed in this paper where individuals continue to refuse to comply with the incentives provided by the state such that low fertility threatens this economic status, Chesnais resorts to the philosophical stance that states are no more than embodiments of the public will: and therefore will not ignore the long-term consequences of low fertility 'unless these consequences are desired by the public'(14).

Although laudable, this proposition side-steps the issue, for in practice certain sectors of the 'public' will invariably support the state's demographic objectives - and recommend measures to achieve them - which will not accord with the wishes of other sectors of that same public which would include the PPA.

By contrast, Van den Brekel does not conform to the position that the state exists to represent the public will, but rather that the state <u>may have to defend itself against this 'will'</u> in the public's own interest:

Freedom of decision (. . . to decide freely with respect to reproduction) must itself be limited; freedom of decision must be constrained by the social duty to act responsibly, and the well-being of society as a whole must be an important criterion.'(15)

While conceding that the 'element of the right of the individual to decide freely often has more weight than the reverse of the coin', he poses the argument that society may have to protect itself against 'hyperindividualisation' where this phenomenon is perceived to threaten the society's future. The argument here is that individuals must choose to temper their own wishes in a sense of social responsibility to the society in which they live, to avoid the 'disruption of social structures'.

As a result of this moral imperative, a number of justifiable avenues of state intervention to influence individual decisions on parenthood are considered:

Coercive policies and pressures must be rejected. Official policies in this field should be restricted to the promotion of knowledge and population consciousness by educational means, by information of campaigns and guidance programmes, supplemented with such socio-economic measures or welfare provisions as are likely to prove incentives towards the desired demographic objective'(16)

Introducing the evaluative concept 'hyper-individualism' into the field of reproductive behaviour would appear to place PPAs in a difficult situation, in the light of their obligation to defend individual freedom to limit births (whatever the demographic-economic forecasts). For it is left to servants of the state to decide when this 'perverse' form of individualism begins to manifest itself and what measures should be used to confront it.

In the light of continuing low fertility, it would be for the PPA, among other representatives of sectional interests, to decide when official 'guidance programmes' as proposed by Van den Brekel, come close to the propaganda that undermines free-choice of which Chesnais warned.

Planned Parenthood Information and Services as the Right of Young People

It has been argued above that, although the prospect of further fertility decline means that PPAs are likely to find it increasingly difficult to persuade governments to extend planned parenthood services, they must endeavour to enlist their support in checking 'violations' of such rights. In no area is this obligation more controversial than that of sex education and contraceptive services for young people. The inclusion of sex/family life education within this project's definition of planned parenthood demands that PPAs distinguish the rights of minors from the traditional rights of the parents to whom those minors 'belong'.

Sex education is qualitatively distinct from other constituents of planned parenthood for, according to what it is desired to teach, it simultaneously defines 'planned parenthood rights' and provides the means by which such rights can be <u>responsibly</u> exercised.

The State has built around the family an elaborate legal structure: it prescribes a minimum age for marriage, and forbids marriage between close relatives; it obliges parents to support offspring through the period when they are unable to fend for themselves and regulates property relations between members. The procreation and rearing of children as a principal function of the family is of interest to others besides parents.

Precisely because children are automatically members of families, having no choice in this matter, and because they are subject to parental authority, their well-being and interests are also partially guaranteed by the State. Equally, other citizens and voluntary associations have an interest in this matter, as it is of general concern that children should be equipped to become sociable and useful men and women.

In Planned Parenthood in the Context of Human Rights, Sjövall extends the logic of the founding pioneers of the IPPF - that women should have the knowledge and means to control their own fertility as a basic human right - to include men and all young people:

Informed, conscious or planned parenthood, taken seriously, really includes all our human rights aspects in the field, from appropriate information to the individual human right to knowledge and means for restricting or promoting fertility at reproductive age.(page 23 above)

Initiatives made during the 1960s by the IPPF included adolescents as special groups at risk in terms of human rights. IPPF policy on 'meeting the needs of young people' (17) states: 'in many situations the right of many people to family planning education and services is denied. FPAs should seek ways of removing legal, administrative and other barriers to the availability of adequate education and services.

In his conclusion, Sjövall seeks to reflect upon the philosophical and psychic basis on which claims to human rights are ultimately founded. He discovers this in the existential desire for personal survival, something which is at least partially guaranteed through parenthood:

Now parenthood happens to have a very profound significance for both these aspects of human survival because on the one hand my child represents the most obvious and concrete manifestation of my material and physical survival and on the other hand the symbolic manifestation of the survival of my identity in terms of being reared and fostered in accordance with my personal value-system.

Granted, therefore, that survival in various existential interpretations of that concept may be considered a universal human right, parenthood has, perhaps, the most obvious and concrete significance in this respect for the predicament of mankind, which places our movement in a very particular and crucial position.

This 'ultimate' justification of human rights to planned parenthood is founded not only on the sense of survival which offspring provide, but, further, through the socialisation of these offspring in the parents' own image. While undoubtedly valid, this appeal harbours serious practical problems for PPAs which are obliged to represent to the state the rights of minors against their parents. Such a dilemma can occur in the area of sex education. The issue Sjövall's justification raises is that the educational rights of young people are subordinate to the existential rights of their parents.

However, the evidence compiled by this project will suggested that the most severe restrictions of planned parenthood rights relate as much to young people's access to sex/contraceptive information and education as to adults' access to contraceptive and related services. Moreover, these restrictions are imposed, in the majority of cultures, by <u>parents</u>, with the complicity of a disinterested or conservative state education system.

Insofar as children are the manifestations of the 'survival of their parents' identity and value-system', they must also sometimes carry the sexual impoverishment or repression of their parents. In many cultures, a repressive sexual socialisation is often defended by the family against the intrusion of the State through formal education.

A PPA must consider the implications of its role on behalf of the rights of young people vis-à-vis their parents on the subject of sexual knowledge. Brodie prescribes a similar role to an organisation such as the US Joint Commission on the Mental Health of Children which is concerned with,

> . . . who protects the child from his protectors, who guards against the guardians, and what mechanisms and which persons provide the best means to gain and protect the rights of children to basic care and self-realisation (and) to acquire the intellectual and emotional skills necessary to achieve individual aspirations and to cope effectively in our society(18)

It is in the field of sex education that the managerial powers of the state can be brought to bear to assist PPAs in their defence of individual rights, though the latter must be ideologically equipped to deal with the conflict in public image which this can present.

Sweden provides an illustration here, though the public image issue is less problematic in that culture because of the high level of social consensus concerning sexual and relationship values. There, this social consensus has been sufficient to permit the State to devise an instruction programme for teachers which is a compulsory part of the curriculum in schools. To those parents who may object on cultural or religious grounds, it is subtly and persuasively argued (akin to Van den Brekel's position) that, if for no other reason, the state must impart certain sexual norms to protect the social system against individual sexual ignorance or destructiveness.(19)

However, the Swedish example is exceptional, at least in Western European states, where governments either feel more comfortable siding with the parent as educator in this field, or, more typically, remaining as uninvolved as possible. It is for the PPA to articulate a convincing rationale for such involvement where necessary.

Conclusion

This paper has attempted to describe ideological dilemmas - described as 'conflicts of obligation' - which arise out of the objectives of planned parenthood associations and their international federation. It has been proposed that as governments have increasingly directed their attention to the role of fertility rates in economic development, these dilemmas are intensified.

For historical and political reasons, there is now widespread support among European governments for the right of individuals to decide for themselves on the number and spacing of children. However, it remains unclear to what extent such individuals will be willing to alter their fertility intentions in the spirit of 'social responsibility' applauded by Van den Brekel to accord with government approaches to attaining longer-term economic targets.

Historically, the prospect of a division of sympathies has been irrelevant to the majority of PPAs, due to the confrontational/campaigning role vis-à-vis states and other authorities in defence of women's health. However, it may reasonably be argued that their success in winning the cooperation of such authorities (to the extent in many cases of becoming dependent upon their financial support) brings with it a quid pro quo of PPA acceptance of the need (if not active support) for policy measures aimed at influencing fertility behaviour in accord with socio-economic planning which has the general support of the population as a whole. For in another context, governments (political parties) prove to be allies in the PPA struggle against other power groups within society (eg. religious and related moral pressure groups which include parents) where it is necessary to defend/promote the rights of weaker sectors of the population such as the young.

If this is so, the further individual fertility decisions deviate from national demographic-economic desiderata, the more complex the PPA relationship with government becomes. As a major donor to government-approved contraceptive services in developing countries, the IPPF's position is similarly complicated by its espousal of the right of individuals ultimately to decide on the number and spacing of children on the one hand, and its recognition of the need for governments' to balance the population-economic equation on the other.

In sum, the European and Third World situations present the planned parenthood movement with similar ideological paradoxes in spite of diametrically opposite fertility trends. In both cases this movement is compelled to direct its information and education activities at both governments and national populations at least with the conviction, if not the certainty, that a convergence of individual fertility desires and nationally-planned economic growth or stability can be achieved.

NOTES

1.   It is also possible to interpret legal restrictions on abortion and lack of adequate contraceptive availability to meet demand as indicative of covert pronatalist intent.

2.   Eversley, D. and Köllmann, W. ed. Population Change and Social Planning 1982 Arnold, London, p. 432.

3.   Yuan Tien, H. 'Changing population policy approaches in China', Intercom 1981 Vol 9, No 10 p. 10.

4.   Ceterchi,I. et al, Law and Population Growth in Romania 1974, Bucharest, pp. 13, 51-58, 284, 293.

5.   For further reading on the early years of the movement see: Suitters, B.: Be Brave and Angry 1973 IPPF pp. 1-19.

6.   Democracy in America, quoted in: Benn, R and Peters, S. Social Principles and the Democratic State 1959 George, Allen & Unwin, London, p. 280.

7.   'Populationist' approaches may be described as taking a different route to the securing of human rights: that is through the arrest of population growth through contraceptive practice as a means to providing the suitable grounds for economic growth; this growth in turn seen as

constituting the optimum conditions for the realisation of human rights.

8. see Van de Kaa, D.J. 'Towards a Population Policy for Western Europe' in Population Decline in Europe, 1978 Council of Europe and; Van den Brekel J.C. 'Population Policy in the Council of Europe Region: Policy Responses to Low Fertility Conditions' European Population Conference.

9. McIntosh, C.A. Population Policy in Western Europe 1983 p. 10 M.E. Sharpe Inc.

10. Chesnais, J-C. 'Fertility and the State' European Population Conference 1982, EPC (82) 14-E Strasbourg.

11. Although feminists may argue that any large-scale financial incentive scheme which aims to induce women to remain at home to bear and rear children would constitute a threat to their chances in the employment market, and therefore their human rights to self-development in the wider community.

12. For example, in the Federal Republic of Germany, a 1977 survey discovered that 21% of couples wanted only one child; 10% said they wished to remain childless. The popularity of childlessness is increasing throughout the developed world - in USA 25% of young women may remain permanently childless. This is of course not to imply that fertility regulation methods and services cause the low fertility trend. However, behavioural changes which have occured would have been unlikely to happen without them. See Family Planning Perspectives 1983 Vol 15 No 5.

13. Chesnais, op cit; Van den Brekel, J.C. Population Policy in the Council of Europe Region: Policy Responses to Low Fertility Conditions, 1982 European Population Conference, EPC (82) 15-E Strasbourg p. 9.

14. op. cit. p. 10

15. Van den Brekel op. cit. p. 11

16. ibid.

17. IPPF Medical Bulletin 1984 Vol 18 No 2 April London.

18. Brodie, E.B. 'Reproductive Freedom, Coercion and Justice' Social Science and Medicine, 1976 Vol 10 p. 555

19. National Swedish Board of Education Instruction Concerning Interpersonal Relations 1977 Liber Utbildningsförlaget, Stockholm, p. 122.

Chapter Four

THE STATUS OF THE HUMAN RIGHT TO PLANNED PARENTHOOD IN INTERNATIONAL RESOLUTIONS

United Nations: A Chronology of Selected Landmarks 1946-84
N Petric

Introduction

In recent times, particularly over the last decade, politicians and social scientists have been forced to confront the issue of the effects of population growth on economic standards, and the measures which might be taken at the UN or similar level to mitigate its negative effects on living standards.

Unfortunately, there is still evidence, in this sphere, of naive correlation between population and economic development in the formulation of 'solutions' particularly to Third World problems. It is necessary to look, rather, to UN statements on the need for changes in existing economic relations as a prerequisite to solutions to global problems, <u>within which</u> the population variable plays only an incidental part. It is unnecessary to restate that population growth per se is not <u>the</u> cause of poverty and under-development; birth control will not alone resolve the problems of the modern developing world. The key lies in pursuit of the New International Economic Order as defined by the UN which is based upon extensive economic cooperation between nations.

The impetus for economic development must stem from national populations themselves, with the necessary incentives and assistance, part of which is the guarantee of the right to freely decide on the number and spacing of the their children. It is with such confidence that these populations will respond to their responsibilities to act for the common good.

Chronology

Historically, UN concern with the human right to decide on the number and spacing of children was preceded by a preoccupation with the population policy aspects of family planning. Only from the mid-60s did a turning point occur when the issue of family planning as such was adopted by the UN as its own and thereafter human rights aspects were overtly discussed in different UN fora.

In 1946 the UN established its **Population Commission** which prepared a two-year work programme. Its analysis identified different population policy approaches: the so-called 'Anglo-Saxon Malthusian'; the 'French pronatalist'; and the 'Eastern European country' approaches.

In the **Universal Declaration of Human Rights,** adopted on 10 December 1948, clause 25 included the statement that 'Maternity and childhood must enjoy particular protection and assistance', which provided a context for family planning.

In 1951, the UN published data an population growth without, however, immediately attracting the attention of demographers and politicians.

In 1954, the **First World Population Conference** was held in Rome under the auspices of the UN and the International Union for the Scientific Study of Population (IUSSP). The subject of 'birth control' was not explicitly discussed at the Conference (although it had been discussed at a World Population Conference held in Zurich in 1927 under League of Nations auspices). Nevertheless, some of the papers delivered referred to family planning eg. 'The Present State of Family Planning among the Peasants and Miners of Japan'; 'The Case for Birth Control in Puerto Rico'. The Conference also heard anti-Malthusian arguments.

During the Conference there emerged a conflict between the representatives from Poland and the USSR, on one side, and those of 'Western' countries on the other. Debate revolved around the interrelationship between population, economic development and social change. It was claimed that the problems of developing countries stemmed not from rapid population growth, but slow economic development resulting from consequences of colonialism. Western representatives (USA, France) insisted that rapid population growth contributed to the slow economic advancement of developing countries. Nevertheless, the neo-Malthusian standpoint did not dominate the Conference, which was regarded as a success by the Socialist countries.

In 1961, a representative of the Swedish government proposed that population problems be discussed at the **UN General Assembly 17th Session** in December 1962. At that meeting the subject was a major topic and resulted in the adoption of a Resolution 'recognising that the health and welfare of the family are of paramount importance, not only for obvious humanitarian reasons, but also with regard to economic development and social progress, and that the health and welfare of the family require special attention in areas with a relatively high rate of population growth'(1838 XVII).

Representatives of Roman Catholic countries had argued against explicit reference to family planning in the Resolution, and the Argentinian delegate had asserted that the UN was not authorised to consider family planning, on the grounds that this would produce moral and political conflicts. The Italian delegate had cited the penalties then in force in his country for promoting contraception. The Spanish delegate declared birth control to be a step towards abortion, euthanasia and other undesirable practices. The Irish delegate asserted that population was not a world problem. On the other hand, the Swedish delegate proposed that population studies be undertaken by governments at national level.

The Resolution was implemented by a UN Economic and Social Council (ECOSOC) Resolution in 1964 in terms of requesting governments to train experts in the field of population (1048 XXXVII). This was followed by a further ECOSOC Resolution in 1965 'considering that there is a need to intensify and extend the scope of the work of the United Nations and the specialised agencies relating to population questions' (1084 XXXIX).

In 1965, at the **18th Session of the UN Commission on the Status of Women,** a Resolution proposed by the representative of the UAR, and supported by representatives from Austria, Finland and USA, was adopted, affirming that 'married couples should have access to all relevant educational information concerning family planning'. The Resolution, using for the first time in the UN the term 'family planning', called for an investigation into the relationship between family planning and the status of women.

Also in 1965, the **18th World Health Assembly Resolution** (18.49) recognised 'that problems of human reproduction involved the family unit as well as society as a whole, and that the size of the family should be the free choice of each individual family'.

In the period between the 1954 First Population

Conference and the 1965 Second Conference, other important discussions on population took place within the UN, including aspects of birth control and equality between women and men. Different development agencies employed the terms 'family planning' and 'birth control' indiscriminately. While differences in approach, reflected in the language used, are now easier to distinguish, terminological problems are yet to be fully overcome.

At the Second World Population Conference, held in Belgrade in 1965, about 800 experts attended from 88 countries, with some 200 observers. The Conference aimed to improve understanding of contemporary demographic processes. Of the 43 authors of papers submitted at the Conference, only 3 were women - an indication of the low profile women had in discussions of their role in society. A meeting, held in parallel to the Conference, and prepared in cooperation with the IPPF and the Yugoslav Federal Council for Family Planning, discussed family planning and agreed the right of couples to decide on the number and spacing of their children.

However, delegates expressed different views on the form which family planning should assume in developing countries. While family planners, notably from Denmark, Mauritius and Yugoslavia, raised the matter of women's rights in developing countries, the Irish delegate formulated a resolution opposing family planning, citing among other arguments the profit motive of contraceptive manufacturers.

In retrospect, 1965 may be seen as a turning point in overcoming resistance to UN involvement in family planning. At the **19th World Health Assembly,** in 1966, a Resolution (19.43) endorsing World Health Organisation (WHO) programme activities in this field referred explicitly to the development of activities 'in family planning, as part of an organised health service'. In December 1966, the UN Secretary General circulated a **Declaration on Population,** signed by 12 Heads of State, which included the statement: 'We believe that the majority of parents wish to acquire the knowledge and means to plan their families . . . to decide on the number and spacing of their children is a basic human right'. This Declaration was subsequently signed by a further 18 Heads of State.

A few days later, the UN General Assembly adopted a Resolution on **Population Growth and Economic Development** 'Recognising the sovereignty of nations in formulating and promoting their own population policies, with due regard to the principle that the size of the family should be the free choice of each individual family'(2211 XXI).

In 1967, the UN established its **Fund for Population Activities (UNFPA),** which has become an important source of financing for population and family planning projects. The fact that the largest donations came from the wealthiest UN member states initially posed problems regarding criteria for allocating UNFPA monies, with some believing that they should be mainly used for developing effective population control measures. In the same year the World Bank made it obligatory for grant-recipient states to report on their demographic trends. In his report in 1968, the World Bank President expressed the view that development aid should be linked to population growth reduction.

The adoption of a Declaration on **Elimination of Discrimination Against Women** by the UN General Assembly in 1967 significantly advanced planned parenthood as a human right in the sense of identifying the right to information and education on family planning and asserting that women have the same rights as men regarding 'access to education and information which contributes to the health and welfare of the family' (2263 XXII).

By 1968, opposition to WHO policy regarding family planning had been largely overcome with the adoption at the **21st World Health Assembly** of Resolution 21.43 which recognised that 'family planning is viewed by many Member States as an important component of basic health services, particularly of maternal and child health and in the promotion of family health and plays a role in social and eocnomic development' and asserted that 'every family should have the opportunity of obtaining information and advice on problems connected with family planning'.

Article 16 of the Proclamation made by the **International Conference on Human Rights,** held in Teheran in 1968, stated that 'Parents have a basic human right to determine freely and responsibly the number and spacing of their children'. This Article was sponsored by the UAR and supported by Chile, Finland, India, Morocoo, Pakistan, Sweden, Turkey and Yugoslavia.

Some disagreement on rights to information in this respect was expressed in drafting the **Declaration on Social Progress and Development,** with objections from Argentina, Brazil, Cuba, Gabon, Nicaragua and Portugal. However, the

Declaration finally adopted by the UN General Assembly 24th Session in December 1969, stated that 'Parents have the exclusive right to determine freely and responsibly the number and spacing of their children', and that 'the construction and implementation according to necessity of a population programme within the context of a national demographic policy as a component of social and medical services includes: the education of service-providers and the creation of conditions to communicate necessary information to families to enable them to exercise their right to determine the number and spacing of children'.

The **Strategy for the Second UN Development Decade,** drafted by the Committee on Development of Planning, and adopted by the General Assembly 25th Session in 1970, reaffirmed the human right to family planning, and stated that 'each developing country should formulate its own demographic objectives within the framework of its development plan'. The responsibility of international organisations to extend appropriate assistance on request was also stated, emphasising that any such assistance was not a substitute for other forms of development assistance.

Preparation for World Population Year 1974 included the organisation in 1972, 1973 and 1974 of UN seminars on human rights aspects of family planning. The **World Population Conference,** held in Bucharest in 1974, differed from the previous two World Conferences in that it was truly intergovernmental. Opinion was divided at the Conference as to whether priority should be given to development or to population-control. Developing country representatives, and those from socialist countries favoured giving priority to development in terms of rapid implementation of the Action Programme of the New International Economic Order. At the same time these countries acknowledged the need to intensify international action contributing to population growth reduction. Thus attempts to treat population/family planning outside the broad scope of socio-economic development were thwarted.

The **World Population Plan of Action** (WPPA) adopted by the World Population Conference included articles on family planning as a human right, notably 14(f): 'All couples and individuals have the basic right to decide freely and responsibly the number and spacing of their children and to have the information, education and means to do so; the responsibility of couples and individuals to exercise this right takes into account the needs of their

children and to have the information, education and means
to do so; the responsibility of couples and individuals to
exercise this right takes into account the needs of their
living and future children, and their responsibilities
towards the community'.

The **UN World Conference of the International Women's
Year** held in Mexico in 1975 also adopted a Plan of Action,
in which Article 12 stated: 'Every couple and every
individual has the right to decide freely and responsibly
whether or not to have children as well as to determine
their number and spacing, and to have information,
education and means to do so'.

Article 19 stated further that: 'Individuals and
couples have the right freely and responsibly to determine
the number and spacing of their children and to have the
information and the means to do so. The exercise of this
right is basic to the attainment of any real equality
between the sexes and without its achievement women are
disadvantaged in their attempt to benefit from other
reforms.'

In 1980, in Copenhagen, the **World Conference of the UN
Mid-Decade for Women (1975-1985) (Equality, Development and
Peace)** reaffirmed the basic human right to family planning
as worded in the 1968 Teheran Proclamation.

The International Development Strategy for the Third
UN Development Decade adopted by the UN General Assembly
in 1981 included the following statement: 'Population
policies will be considered as an integral part of overall
development policies. All countries will continue to
integrate their population measures and programmes into
their social and economic goals and strategies. Within the
framework of national demographic policies, countries will
take the measures they deem necessary concerning fertility
levels in full respect of the right of parents to determine
in a free, informed and responsible manner the number and
spacing of their children. The international community
will increase the level of population assistance in support
of those measures. In addition, due consideration should
be given to the need for increased biomedical and social
science research into safer, more efficient and more widely
acceptable techniques of fertility regulation.'

In anticipation of the World Population Conference,
the United Nations' **Economic Commission for Europe** held a
meeting on population in Bulgaria in 1983, 'to provide a
forum for governments of the ECE Region to discuss and

exchange views . . . (and) . . . to formulate suggestions and recommendations for further implementation of the World Population Plan of Action.' The following were among recommendations forthcoming:

Governments should incorporate into population policies the principle that it is a fundamental right of couples and individuals to decide freely and responsibly the number and spacing of their children by formulating measures and regulations, including those concerning fertility control, consistent with this right. Couples and individuals should be assured of the means, information and education to plan their families in accordance with this principle. (Recommendation 32)

Education, medical and legal provisions should be made to assist couples and individuals to avoid unwanted pregnancies. The necessary measures should be taken, including those governing the availability of safe and effective methods of birth control, together with medical consultations, counselling and sex education, particularly among those segments of the populatiuon which are most vulnerable and difficult to reach. In view of the increased incidence of sexual relationships among adolescents and the lower age at which sexual experience begins, special attention, notably in the form of family life and sex education and of medical services for young people, should be given to avoid unplanned and unwanted pregnancies of adolescents for health as well as socio-economic reasons. (Recommendation 37)

The **International Conference on Population** met in **Mexico City** in August 1984 to appraise the implementation of the World Population Plan of Action, adopted by consensus in Bucharest ten years previously. The Conference reaffirmed the full validity of the principles and objectives of the World Plan, adopting a set of recommendations for further implementation which included the following:

Recommendation 26: 'Governments should, as a matter of urgency, make universally available information, education and the means to assist couples and individuals to achieve their desired number of children. Family planning information, education and means should include all medically approved and appropriate methods of family planning, including natural family planning, to ensure a voluntary and free choice in accordance with changing individual and cultural values. Particular attention should be given to those segments of the population which are most vulnerable and difficult to reach.'

Recommendation 30: 'Governments are urged to ensure that all couples and individuals have the basic right to decide freely and responsibly the number and spacing of their children and to have the information, education and means to do so; the responsibility of couples and individuals in the exercise of this right takes into account the needs of their living and future children and their responsibilities towards the community.'

Recommendation 31: 'Legislation and policies concerning the family and programmes of incentives and disincentives should be neither coercive nor discriminatory and should be consistent with internationally recognised human rights as well as with changing individual and cultural values.'

Recognising the potential antagonism between national population policies and the free exercise of individual rights to determine fertility, Recommendation 13 states: 'Countries which consider that their population growth rates hinder the attainment of national goals are invited to consider pursuing relevant demographic policies within the framework of socio-economic development. Such policies should respect human rights, the religious beliefs, philosophical convictions, cultural values and fundamental rights of each individual and couple, to determine the size of its own family.'

This is reaffirmed within Recommendations 33: 'Governments that have adopted or intend to adopt fertility policies are urged to set their own quantitative targets in this area. Countries implementing family planning programmes should establish programme targets at the operational level, respecting the basic right of couples and individuals to decide freely and responsibly the number and spacing of their children, taking into account the needs of their living and future children and their responsibilities, exercised freely and without coercion towards the community.' And Recommendation 35: 'Governments that view the level of fertility in their countries as to low may consider financial and other support to families to assist them with their parental responsibilities and to facilitate their access to the necessary services. Such policies should not restrict access to education, information and services for family planning.'

Council of Europe Resolutions on Family Planning

Following the European Population Conference, organised in 1971, the Council of Europe Committee of Ministers responded to one of the Conference recommendations by establishing an intergovernmental Committee of Experts now known as the Steering Committee on Population (CDDE), on which the IPPF Europe Region enjoys observer status.

The Steering Committee considers that the results of demographic studies do not usually lend themselves to formulation in terms of a quasi-legal instrument such as a recommendation of the Committee of Ministers to the governments of member states. In most cases, it is the role of demographers to contribute their specialist insights to the policy-making process rather than proposing policies themselves, population usually being one factor among many which have to be taken into account in any particular area of policy formulation.

There has been one exception to this practice so far. As a result of work by the former Committee of Demographic Experts, the Committee of Ministers adopted Resolution (75) 29 on legislation relating to fertilty and family planning. This resolution was an attempt to translate into policy terms at the European level the principle reaffirmed in the 1974 World Population Plan of Action that 'all couples and individuals have the right to decide freely and responsibly the number and spacing of their children· It sets out guidelines for governments in the following areas: family planning services, education in family planning, sterilisation, abortion and economic and social assistance to families. (See Appendix 1).

Following work by the European Health Committee (CDSP), the Committee of Ministers further adopted Resolution (78)10 on Family Planning Programmes (See Appendix 1).

At the 1982 European Population Conference one of the Conclusions adopted (no. 10) contained the following statement: 'In a democratic society, the right of individual men and women to decide freely and responsibly on the number and spacing of their children should be regarded as fundamental and deserves priority above all other considerations. Amongst other things, this implies that free access to family planning services should be assured so as to implement the Resolutions on family planning adopted by the Council of Europe in 1975 and 1978.'

Following the Conference, the Committee of Ministers invited governments of Council of Europe Member States* to report on implementation of the two Resolutions. By the beginning of 1985 about half of the Member States had reported. The reports are expected to become available later in 1985.

---

*MEMBER STATES: Austria, Belgium, Cyprus, Denmark, France, Federal Republic of Germany, Greece, Iceland, Ireland, Italy, Liechtenstein, Luxembourg, Malta, Netherlands, Norway, Portugal, Spain, Sweden, Switzerland, Turkey, United Kingdom.

Chapter Five

NATIONAL PROFILES

ISSUES:

1   Government recognition of the human right to determine the number and spacing of children, within the context of its responsibilities for protection of family and child.

2   Family planning facilities/services. (Government and other)

3   The sale, distribution and advertisement of contraceptives.

4   The availability/sale of family planning-related literature.

5   Sterilisation.

6   Abortion.

7   Infertility treatment.

8   Sex education/family life education.

9   Adoption.

The data that follows was collected during 1984.

Issue	De Jure	De Facto
1. Government recognition of human right to number and spacing of children (planned parenthood)	The individual right to the free determination of number and spacing of children is implied in the Constitution.	With the exception of Government provision of facilities for sterilization, abortion, and general services for adolescents, the de jure situation is well reflected in practice.
Protection of family and child.	There are a number of federal laws containing provisions on economic and social assistance to families.	
2. Government and other family planning (fp) facilities/services.	There is no legislation covering government family planning facilities. A law exists permitting advertisement of family planning clinics.	All Government clinic services are free of charge (167 clinics), and practically all GPs provide some family planning service. However, the standards of these are neither monitored nor controlled. Government services exist as part of hospitals, Mother and Child Health (MCH) care and other centres. They offer specialised services for adolescents, migrants and women only. There are no marked differences between urban and rural areas except for IUD and sterilisation availability. Government training for personnel. Clinics are publicised via national and local authority produced leaflets as dictated by national policy Counselling is also available in Government-funded centres. Private family planning services exist independently of State services.
3. The sale, distribution and advertisement of contraceptives.	With the exception of the oral contraceptive, the sale/distribution of contraceptives is not prohibited by law. Orals are considered as medicines and therefore subject to the Drug Act. Their advertisement is legally permitted.	Contraceptives are not supplied free of charge through the State services. Condoms are advertised and available in pharmacies and condom vending machines also exist. There are no practical obstacles to obtaining contraceptives except for adolescents who may not be welcomed by all physicians.
4. Availability/sale of family planning (fp) related literature	No law exists covering the sale of fp related literature.	Since there is no law to prohibit the sale/availability of fp related literature, it is widely available in book-shops, fp clinics etc. Literature appears in crie de coeur ('agony aunt') letters in newspapers, books and leaflets, most of it produced commercially. Depending on its nature, it may be obtained from bookshops, and is enclosed in packaging of tampons.

Issue	De Jure	De Facto
5. Sterilisation	Sterilisation is legally regulated as a method of family planning in the following terms: 'Sterilisation performed by a medical doctor is not illegal if the patient consents, and provided that the latter is over 25 years old, or if such a practice is not contrary to good practice if performed on other grounds'.	Although sterilisation is permitted, it is not a preferred method and physicians usually try to persuade clients to postpone it until after their 35th year (women). Vasectomies are more difficult to obtain because of the reluctance of the medical profession to perform them (due to fear of clients' change of mind after the event), and a general lack of interest by the male population.
		Most sterilisations are paid for through health insurance 'under cover' of other medically necessary surgery. The number of sterilisations performed annually is unknown as no law requires the keeping of such records. Moreover, private physicians may perform sterilisations.
6. Abortion	Decriminalisation of abortion was achieved in the 1970s. Induced abortion was legalised after 1975 up to the first trimester on any grounds - providing the woman consented to the termination and had received appropriate counselling by medically qualified personnel. On certain medical grounds abortions may be performed within the law beyond the first trimester. Induced abortion is not paid for by (normal) health insurance, nor is it subject to obligatory notification.	Due to conscientious objection from medical personnel and hospital management, abortion facilities are not readily available all over the country.
		Abortions are not performed free of charge in State premises.
		In view of the legal situation prevailing today, it is not believed that illegal abortion is practised on any scale.
	These regulations also apply to minors.	There is no legal requirement to record the number of abortions performed so statistics are not available. It is permitted to advertise abortion in newspapers.
7. Infertility treatment	Infertility treatment and artificial insemination are not legally regulated.	Some specialised hospitals and private physicians provide artificial insemination, though the service is not widely available throughout the country.
		While infertility treatment in general is covered by health insurance, artificial insemination must be paid for privately.
		The level of demand for AID/AIH (donor/husband) is unknown.

Issue	De Jure	De Facto
8. Sex education/family life education	Sex education is legally regulated as part of the school curriculum and it is theoretically implemented in elementary, secondary, and higher education levels. The instruction of the Federal Ministry of Education and Arts (Jan 1st 1971) points to the importance of contacts between school and parents.	The situation is not reflected in practice, though some sex education is available in some schools according to the willingness of the teaching staff.
		The mass media regularly feature sex education.
9. Adoption	The reform of family legislation in 1960 resulted in a new understanding of the essence and spirit of adoption. The well-being of the minors to be adopted is regarded as the most important consideration. The adoption may take place based on a court writ. The law specifies the age requirement of adopters. The law also recognises 'incognito' adoption, where the names and residence of the adopters remain confidential. Adopted children take on the rights of natural born children.	While demand appears to be stable, there are too few children available for the numbers wishing to adopt. However, foster children cannot easily find foster parents in spite of a new law giving such parents greater rights.
	Minimum ages for adopters are set at 28 for mother and 30 for father.	

Issue	De Jure	De Facto
1. Government recognition of human right to number and spacing of children (planned parenthood)	In general, the law codifying family life, procreation and sexuality is based on the ideas laid down in the Code Napoleon (The Penal Code dates from 1867, later adapted but up to now, not fundamentally revised). For example, it is not basically adapted to the profound disassociation of procreation from sexuality, which evolved during this century. The emphasis remains on the protection of the family; emphasis favours marriage and discriminates against patterns of sexuality which exclude procreation. This subject is not regarded as a priority by the Government, but rather left to the private sector (incl. medical profession) for the provision of services.	No explicit or direct promotion of planned parenthood as a basic human right. The only effort made by the Government in this field was a 'Responsible Parenthood' campaign in 1974, which comprised the production and distribution of a booklet for paramedical staff and social workers, and a brochure for the public. For this, a special budget of Belgian Francs 25 million was set aside. This could be regarded as a rather inconsequential and arbitrary initiative which was intended mainly to distract from the abortion debate in the country (1971-73). Throughout the years, the Government has assisted in this field through its subsidies to counselling centres concerned, in part, with fertility regulation problems.
2. Government and other family planning (fp) facilities/services		Government fp services do not exist; i.e. family planning is conducted solely by non-governmental/private organisations.
3. The sale, distribution and advertisement of contraceptives	The sale of contraceptives and contraceptive literature is not legally forbidden. The distribution of contraceptives is legally regulated. A Law of July 1973 permits contraceptive advertising though restrictions remain on 'medicaments'. Fp consumer literature is readily available through: fp clinics, bookshops and libraries.	Condoms are sold in pharmacies and other shops. Orals are sold in pharmacies on prescription only. It has become more difficult to obtain the diaphragm. During the 1970s, and after the law of 1973; a number of organisations (Women's Movement, Consumer Organisation), the Family Movement Association etc) either produced leaflets or published articles on contraception to inform their members on the subject. Since this time all organisations have become complacent, presuming that sufficient information is now available. The Belgian PPA alone continues to provide information for groups in need such as adolescents; and to inform the public about sterilisation, AID etc.

Issue	De Jure	De Facto
3. The sale, distribution and advertisement of contraceptives (cont'd)		Only recently have condoms been advertised – on billboards – in Belgium. Contraceptives remain rather expensive for some social groups: adolescents, migrants.
4. Availability/sale of family planning (fp) related literature	No legal impediments	Such literature is available through a variety of outlets (bookshops, fp centres, some youth clubs) though without a high profile (see issue 3).
5. Sterilisation	There is no law covering sterilisation per se. However, the Penal Code of 1867 stipulates penalties for deliberately inflicting wounds on another – which could be used in such cases.	Sterilisation was available initially through obstetrics/gynaecology departments of university medical schools. The service was gradually also provided by private practice gynaecologists (at first, a restricted number known to 'insiders'). By the end of the 1970s, the demand for, particularly, female sterilisation grew, leading to a relaxing of the conditions for eligibility (by the medical profession). Nevertheless, obstacles remain for groups such as the childless, the young, and unmarried. Most sterilisations are now performed in hospitals. Officially the operation must be paid for, though in practice it may be reimbursed through the social security system if medical personnel choose to define it in other medical terms.
6. Abortion	The law forbids abortion on any grounds. The advertisement of abortion services is prohibited.	In practice, abortions have been performed to date for morally defensible medical/psychological reasons. Operations have been registered and addresses of facilities publicised. In contrast, judicial authorities in the Brussels area have, in the 1980s, initiated prosecutions against medical personnel involved in abortion. Parliamentary initiatives to change the prohibitive law remain blocked. Surveys indicate that over 60% of the Belgian people would favour a more liberal law, though the conditions pertaining to such a law may, in practice, produce greater restrictions than exist, de facto, at present.

Issue	De Jure	De Facto
7. Infertility treatment	Not dealt with explicitly by law.	Because of a resolution of the Committee of Ministers of the Council of Europe (1979), Belgian legislators are becoming increasingly sympathetic to 'enabling' laws designed to cover AID etc. In practice AID is provided in the highly specialised university obstetric and gynaecological units. Fp centres, among others, will refer to these units, after counselling.
8. Sex education/family life education (SE/FLE)	This subject is not included in the school curriculum by Government provision.	Sex education is available, through some schools sympathetic to the subject; through adult education classes, youth clubs, and via the mass media. The non-inclusion of SE/FLE in the school curriculum by Government provision can be related to the value-based character of such instruction, and the divisions in the Belgian school system (so-called 'Free' or Catholic schools, and 'State' or official ones). If SE components appear, they will most likely be attached to biology or ethics classes. Although there is little survey evidence on the subject, it is likely that SE is becoming more widespread. For example, sexuality and fertility regulation are components of 'Learning to live and communicate with each other' courses designed for young people.
9. Adoption	Law of March 1969 changed the previous legislation by giving the adopted child the same rights as a natural born child. Conditions: the adopting couple must be a minimum of 30 years of age or at least one partner if the marriage has five years duration. If the adopter is single, he/she must be minimum 35 years of age, and 15 years older than the adoptee.	Demand appears to be increasing even though there are too few children to satisfy demand (particularly newborn, healthy Belgian children). A number of private organisations provide adoption services, though these are costly, time-consuming, and somewhat ideologically biased. Some fp centres have been involved in this area.

Issue	De Jure	De Facto
1. Government recognition of human right to number and spacing of children (planned parenthood)	The right of an individual to free determination of the number and spacing of children is not legally regulated.	The de jure situation is reflected in practice.
Protection of family and child	The protection of family and child is covered by a special family law, and indirectly through other laws and regulations.	
2. Government and other family planning (fp) facilities/services	Family planning facilities/services are legally regulated by Act No. 282, 1972, and followed up and explained in Government Circular March 1976.	There are 24 clinics in Denmark including 2 private clinics, which the Danish PPA, as a non-Governmental organisation, runs in the metropolitan area. The FPA is reimbursed almost in full for this activity by the Municipality and County of Copenhagen.
	Family planning services are available from general practitioners, at hospitals and at special clinics.	According to the Act each county has to establish clinics, and these clinics should also serve as places of education (general practitioners) and research regarding contraception. These purposes have not been met in full in practice.
	Family planning counselling is free of charge, but the consumers have to pay for the contraceptives.	
	The law allows for the advertisement of family planning clinics.	According to Act No. 236, May 1984, concerning pregnancy hygiene and maternity care, it was established that counties are obliged to provide clinics (or hospital wards) as alternative venues for contraception.
3. The sale, distribution and advertisement of contraceptives	There is no legal prohibition of the sale of contraceptives, but the sale/ distribution are legally regulated.	Contraceptives are free-of-charge only on a trial basis in certain counties.
	Oral contraceptives and IUDs are covered by Medicines Act No. 327, 1975, and are sold on prescription only, through pharmacies and fp clinics.	
	There is no legal age limit on the right to receive fp information from clinics/ physicians (i.e. they can be advised without the consent of a guardian/ parent).	
	Condoms and diaphragms are exempt from the Medicines Act and covered by Government Circular No. 81, 1979, and according to which the National Health Service may decide that a contraceptive of another kind may be exempted from the Medicines Act, which has been the case in respect of spermicides.	

Issue	De Jure	De Facto
	Sale and distribution of condoms, diaphragms and spermicides is only permitted on condition that they have been approved by the national health service. Both the Act and Government circular allow for the advertisement of contraceptives. The rules in the act governing advertisement are stricter than those in the circular.	
4. Availability/sale of family planning (fp) related literature.	The sale of fp related literature is not legally regulated.	There are no limitations to the publication and sale of fp related literature. The Danish PPA and other organisations have been given the responsibility by the Ministry of the Interior for provision of appropriate information material to professionals and the public.
5. Sterilisation	Sterilisation is legally regulated, permissible as a method of fp for men and women over the age of 25. (Act No. 318 1973) If a woman is under 25 years of age sterilisation may be performed if it is necessary to avoid pregnancy or to avert danger to the women's life or grave deterioration in her mental/physical health. In these cases, the woman's spouse (legal or not) being under age 25, may be sterilised. This permission can be obtained on grounds of: hereditary predisposition to endanger physical/mental health of potential offspring; inability to care for potential children because of serious mental/physical illness/disability; genetic deficiency of all potential offspring; and socio-economic grounds.	The de jure situation is reflected in practice. Sterilisation takes place only in public hospitals. However, some male sterilisations are performed in outpatient departments.
6. Abortion	Induced abortion is legally regulated by Act No. 350, 1973 which permits abortion on request to any woman resident in Denmark up to the first trimester. After the 12th week, abortion can be performed without special permission if this is necessary to avoid threat to the woman's life or to avoid serious harm to her mental or physical heatlh - if this danger is principally medical. After the first trimester, permission must be (contd).	The de jure situation is reflected in practice. The local hospitals are under an obligation to receive all women wanting abortion up to the first trimester.

Issue	De Jure	De Facto
6. Abortion (contd).	applied for when: the pregnancy/birth would endanger the woman's health – this would include consideration of the woman's living conditions/socio-economic condition; whether the pregnancy was the result of rape; mental physical disease of the embryo; mental capacity of mother to care for offspring; incapacity to care for offspring due to immaturity.	
7. Infertility treatment	At present there are no legal regulations covering this subject but all medical facilities are available.	AID is only performed in public hospitals.
8. Sex education/family life education	Sex education in primary school is legally regulated by Act No. 235, 1970, as an integrated part of the school curriculum. Within the limits of the law the school itself also has a say in what is taught and how this is taught.	In practice it is included in nursery school, elementary school, secondary and higher education. It is felt that the level/quality of provision can yet be improved.
9. Adoption	Adoption is legally regulated by Act No. 272 1972 which makes heavy demands on the potential adoptive parents.	Liberalisation of the Act is at present under review in the Ministry of Justice. In practice only foreign children are available for adoption.

Issue	De Jure	De Facto
1. Government recognition of human right to number and spacing of children (planned parenthood)	The right of an individual to the free determination of the number and spacing of children is not legally regulated, though officially adopted by the Federal Government. The Federal Government's standpoint (1977) is that conditions should be created to facilitate a couple's desire for children.	The present Federal Government, led by the Conservative Party (CUD/CSU) since 1982, shows a tendency toward a pronatalist point of view and a general orientation of its family politics to what is seen as required to suit population and labour market developments.
	By the Supreme Court's decision on the 1974 abortion act (1975) the Federal Government was urged to take measures in support of fertility regulation to prevent unwanted pregnancies and abortions.	Due to the economic climate the present Federal Government has slowed its efforts to meet recognised needs for more specified fp facilities and services initiated by the Social Democratic Party in the late 1970s.
	The Constitutional Law (the central legislative act in the FRG) holds to the principle that marriage and the family enjoy the special protection of the State. It further recognises the natural right of the parents both to look after and to educate their children. This includes recognition of the rights of single-parent families and of the differences in the chosen manner of childbearing, rearing and education.	There are some regulations such as the maternal protection act and transfer of income from single persons to married couples and families which may be seen as implementing the constitutional principles. However, these regulations tend to favour married rather than unmarried couples and single persons with children. Disadvantages increase according to the number of children. Legislation generally favours married against unmarried or single parents.
		Though the present Federal Government emphasizes broader and more effective support of the family (including single-parent families), in fact, there has been a decrease in family-related benefits continuing since the late 1970s e.g. public subsidy for mothers during four months after end of the protection period, which was introduced for women employed before the birth of the child, 'as a first step' in the 70s, is to be reduced by 1984. Government recently proclaimed extension to all mothers by 1987, 'if the financial situation of the State then allows'.
		With regard to the other topics see 2., 4. and 8.

Issue	De Jure	De Facto
2. Family Planning Facilities/Services	Family planning facilities and services are legally regulated in two ways: The statutory health insurance system provides free advice and, if necessary, medical examination and prescription of fertility regulation drugs by physicians and free sterilisation including hospital treatment. Laws and other regulations govern the recognition and financial support of family planning advice services offered by private organisations and ensure that if they fail in establishing them, public services replace them. In most states fp advice is seen as component of marriage guidance and family counselling offices (which are supported to a lesser degree), as well as being the concern of pregnancy and abortion counselling offices (whose public financial support is usually higher).	Private family planning facilities are predominant, and among them services through GPs and gynaecologists' offices play the main role, followed by private fp counselling organisations (mainly Pro Familia) and a small number of family planning clinics. Public counselling facilities exist in most federal states. However, they are visited only by a minority of clients. Public services, only, play a major role in sterilisation (see 5). It is not known to what extent GP's and gynaecologists' offices actually supply fp services. In Berlin, it was reported, only 150 out of 700 authorised physicians had accounted for such services with the statutory health insurance bodies in 1981; this figure, however, may be incomplete. Differences in actual supply between rural and urban areas are probable, but are not quantified. Different indices lead to the conclusion that, with regard to quality, GP's and gynaecologists' fp services are of an unsatisfactory standard. It is believed that this is due to lack of training, to the fact that physicians' training still almost completely neglects counselling abilities, and the lack of sufficient incentives through fees paid by health insurances for such services. Considerable regional differences exist in the distribution of the fp counselling office. e.g. in Bavaria (over 10 million population) there are only 5 compared to more than 20 such offices in Hessen (5,5 million population). In general, in rural areas fp counselling offices are scarcer.
	The advertising of family planning facilities and services is not legally regulated. However, physicians are obliged not to advertise their service to the public in any way.	Actual restriction of advertisements for fp services are not known. Information on available fp counselling services is most frequently to be found in newspapers; in other mass media only occasionally, within reports or features on the subject of fp or abortion.

- 71 -

Issue	De Jure	De Facto
2. Family planning facilities/services (contd).		Leaflets giving information on fp facilities and/or services, which are produced mainly by health insurances, the Federal office for Health Education and Pro Familia, are distributed through GP's offices, hospitals, public health offices etc. Occasionally fp facilities and/or services are advertised in public places or at public fairs and by literature (pocket books) dealing with family planning related subjects.

Special services/facilities: On a local level there are some special fp services addressed to young people, migrants handicapped persons and other groups. Though little is known of the experiences and the effectiveness of such services, they seem to be suitable particularly for migrants (because of communication problems in general services).

Pro Familia is, at present, trying to build up a postcoital treatment service in co-operation with GPs and hospitals.

While GPs and gynaecologists play a main role in fp services, their training is considered inadequate with regard to most aspects of fp related knowledge and counselling.

With the exception of work in counselling centres the participation of other relevant professions such as midwives or social workers is not well developed.

Counselling centres, on the other hand, seem not to be very successful in reaching some population groups, e.g. the lower classes and inhabitants of rural communities.

Fp related research is widely neglected by the Federal Government and is carried out only by commercially interested corporations.

General discussion on fp topics in the public is largely limited to the aspect of abortion avoidance. In this context, there are signs that the present Federal Government led by the conservative CDU/CSU is lending an ear to advice from the Roman Catholic Church to strenthen support for the 'natural' methods. |

Issue	De Jure	De Facto
3. The sale, distribution and advertisement of contraceptives	As there is no legislation on fp as such, the sale, distribution and advertisement of contraceptives is not legally regulated, but by laws and other regulations concerning drugs and medical treatment in general exist.	Pro Familia has taken an initiative to improve public financial support of fp counselling services and to build up more fp clinics. Prospects, however, are estimated not to be very promising at present.
	As a consequence of the 1974/6 abortion legislation, counselling, medical examination and prescription of contraceptives (where carried out by a physician) are free as part of statutory health insurance. In general, consumers have to pay for their contraceptives and any other contraceptive treatment (except sterilisation).	
	Contraceptives and contraceptive treatment are free through doctors and are sold only in pharmacies.	Only a minority of those entitled to claim seem to do so.
	Pills (including post-coital pills) have to be prescribed by doctors and are sold in pharmacies.	This is widely reflected in practice though to some extent doctors distribute pill samples gratis.
	Only physicians may insert IUDs or administer injectables (the latter having been banned recently for normal use by Federal Health Office).	
	Condom vending machines may not be sited in public places, with the exception of restaurants, WCs, etc accessible to the public.	Only physicians may fit diaphragms. Diaphragms, condoms and foam are sold in pharmacies and drug-stores, condoms in vending machines and condoms and foams by mail-order, too.

- 73 -

Issue	De Jure	De Facto
	Commercial advertising of contraceptives is legally regulated only for those regarded as drugs or remedies (pill, IUD). These may be advertised only in the professional press.	Legislation is followed in practice.
	Other commercial advertising is limited only by the general regulations of the civil law (e.g. it is forbidden to advertise a product comparing it with other products or to advertise in a way regarded as obscene).	Commercial advertising in mass media (mainly newspapers and magazines) is common only for foams. Advertising for condoms occurs in magazines.
		Information on all methods is usual through features on fp, abortion and related topics in the mass media and through leaflets on fp distributed in GP's offices, health offices, hospitals, counselling offices etc.
4. Availability/sale of family planning (fp) related literature	No legislation governs the advertisement, sale and dissemination of fp related literature as such.	
	All this, however, is affected by general legislation or other regulations in the following respects:	
	a) Advertising and any kind of distribution making a book available to minors is forbidden when its content is deemed to be pornographic by a court.	Occasionally fp-related literature is banned by a court for reason of pornographic content. Such decisions, however, are not always followed by legal authorities in other court districts.
	b) Teaching books which are free for students at state schools are to be authorised by federal states' governments.	Particularly conservative Governments tend to use this right to influence the content of such literature extensively.
	Federal Government has to authorise literature (leaflets etc.) supported financially by a Government department.	In general, there are no essential problems in this respect. The lack of special legal regulations is regarded as an advantage. However, the availability of fp-related literature depends to a certain degree on the political atmosphere, which has tended to be rather conservative recently.

Issue	De Jure	De Facto
5. Sterilisation	There is no law governing sterilisation as such. Following its legal classification as bodily injury it is generally considered a permitted method of contraception (as injury is not punishable unless it violates 'common practice').	The Federal Board of Physicians (Bundesärztekammer) states that sterilisation should be carried out only when indicated medically or socially. This is interpreted widely in practice.
	As a result of the 1974/76 abortion legislation, counselling and surgical treatment are free for members of the statutory health insurance system (around 90% of population).	However, sterilisation is performed on a rather small scale. Statistical data on this subject are lacking, but it is estimated that no more than around 50,000 sterilisations are carried out each year, the vast majority of them on women
		This seems to be due mainly to:
		a) historical grounds (misuse of sterilisation under Nazi regime);
		b) cautious attitudes among surgeons caused by legal uncertainty (risk of damage claims resulting from failures and doubts remaining on what should be regarded as 'social' indication for sterilisation).
6. Abortion	Induced abortion is legally regulated by a 1976 law (which replaced a more liberal 1974 law denied by Supreme Court in 1975).	Of the 91,000 abortions reported (incomplete), 19% were performed on medical grounds, 2.5% on eugenic, and 77% on social-psychological grounds.
	This states that abortions may be performed:	
	a) on medical grounds (including such that might affect the health of the woman after birth) irrespective of duration of the pregnancy; b) on eugenic grounds up to 22 weeks; c) on social/psychological grounds up to 12 weeks.	
	The law specifies that a physician (not the one carrying out the abortion) must present his decision on the permissibility of the abortion in written form.	Physicians are increasingly sympathetic to requests for abortions, GP's more so than gynaecologists.
	The physician who is to carry out the abortion has to reconsider the legality of the abortion and can reject the decision of the first doctor. No physician is obliged to carry out an	Abortions to be performed on social-psychological grounds are rejected by the heads of some hospitals.

Issue	De Jure	De Facto
	Permissible abortions may be carried out in any hospital and in other state facilities licensed by the state (GPs' and gynaecologists' clinics under certain conditions, and outpatient clinics).	The number of public and private hospitals in which abortions are available varies widely from state to state (see above). In some regions private and/or public hospitals refuse any non medically-grounded abortion (using very strict medical criteria).
		From the abortions reported to the Federal Statistical Office in 1982, 56% were performed in hospitals (4% out-patient) and 44% in other facilities, mainly in GP/gynaecological clinics (all out-patient). The frequency of abortions in hospitals has decreased since 1976.
	Clients must undergo counselling and be informed on the medical aspects of abortion and the availability of private and public assistance should she decide to continue the pregnancy.	
	Following the 1975 Supreme Court decision the counsellor is obliged to try to influence the client's continued pregnancy.	
	Abortion is free for members of the statutory health insurance system (90% of population), if legal conditions are fulfilled. Private health insurance systems re-imburse expenses only for abortions on medical or genetic grounds.	It is estimated that per year in the FRG 130,000 - 150,000 abortions are performed, plus 20,000 - 25,000 abroad (mostly in the Netherlands).
7. Infertility treatment	There is no legislation on infertility treatment as such. Medical examination and counselling by doctor are free for members of the statutory health insurance but not the treatment itself unless it may be regarded as curative treatment, e.g. in the sense, that infertility may be caused by psychological problems.	Infertility treatment may be performed by any approved gynaecologist in university hospitals and private clinics. In fact, there are estimated to be around 20 facilities in the FRG, most of them gynaecologists' clinics, some university hospitals and a few private clinics. However, it is difficult to find an easy-to-reach facility.
		The level of demand is not known.

Issue	De Jure	De Facto
8. Sex education/family life education	Sex education is included in the general school curriculum under regulations of the federal states' governments. Teachers are instructed to combine sex education topics with contents of any related course (such as biology, literature etc.)	In the main, sex education is performed only in biology classes, and there only rather superficially. This is due mainly to the constitutional law which gives parents authority to decide on the nature of sex education provided.
		Sex education is, with a few exceptions, not part of the university training programmes for teachers. There are only a few ongoing training programmes on sex education for teachers working at school, and these are poorly attended.
		Extra-school sex education is offered in some youth clubs. Publications on the subject are widely available to all age groups; however, attempts have been made by governments and legal authorities to influence the contents.
9. Adoption	Adoption is regulated by two laws (both from 1977). One refers to the requirements of recognised adoption agencies. The other refers to the conditions, rights and responsibilities of adopters and adoptees.	The 1977 adoption legislation is commonly regarded as a considerable step forward compared with the former adoption law. Each year there are around 10,000 adoptions while the demand by potential adopters is estimated at 15,000.
		Most problems result from the fact that it is hard to find people ready and qualified to adopt handicapped children. The Federal Government has announced that it will reduce the legal minimum period for parental consent to adoption after birth from the present 8 weeks to 6 in order 'to facilitate adoptions instead of abortions'. Extra financial assistance is to be provided to this end.

Issue	De Jure	De Facto
1. Government recognition of human right to number and spacing of children (planned parenthood)	The right of an individual to the free determination of the number and spacing of children is legally regulated within the terms of the Primary Health Care Act 1966/72. It is expressed as follows. The national Board of Health is obliged, 'to help people in their efforts to avoid unwanted pregnancies; to help to space the pregnancies according to their wishes; to lessen the need for abortion by effective contraception'.	The de jure situation is well reflected through Government practice via the national health system.
Protection of family and child	Protection of family and child is guaranteed indirectly through a variety of legislation: Primary Health Care Act; Employment Act; Child Support Act etc.	
2. Government and other family planning (fp) facilities/services	Family planning is legally regulated (see below). No law forbids the giving of advice on contraception.	FP is available through separate clinics and hospitals. There are no specialised services (available to women only, adolescents only etc.) In addition, the Finnish Population and Family Welfare Federation runs its own specialist clinics for marital and sexual counselling services.

Through the National Health Service the first three months of the pill and first IUD are free, subsequent supplies must be paid for. |
| 3. The sale, distribution and advertisement of contraceptives | No law prohibits the sale of contraceptives or related literature. No law prohibits the production or import of contraceptives for personal use, with the exception of oral contraceptives. Production of the latter requires the permission of the Ministry of Social Affairs and Health. With the exception of oral contraceptives - which may be distributed only with the permission of the National Board of Health (eg. through pharmacies) all contraceptives may be purchased anywhere, including automatic vending machines. Oral contraceptives are available only on a physician's prescription.

No law prohibits the advertisement of contraceptives nor where such advertising may take place. | |
| 4. Availability/sale of family planning (fp) related literature. | There is nothing in the law which prohibits the sale or dissemination of fp related literature. | Consumer literature is readily available through fp clinics, bookshops, libraries, hospitals, health centres, schools and within the armed forces. |

Issue	De Jure	De Facto
5. Sterilisation	Sterilisation is regulated by a law of 1985, made available either: to those (men or women) 30+ years on request; to those with 3 children on request; or to those not fulfilling the above criteria on a decision of two physicians that contraception would not be possible by any other means. It must be performed on licenced premises by appropriate qualified personnel. Spousal consent is not required, though that person must be informed.	
6. Abortion	Induced abortion is legally regulated. It may be performed up to the 12th week of pregnancy on socio-economic grounds. It may not be performed after the 12th week on any grounds other than a disease or physical defect in the woman. (It may be performed between 12-20 weeks on special permission of the State Medical Board.) In most cases, termination of pregnancy needs either the recommendation of two physicians or the authorisation of the State Medical Board and must be performed in approved hospitals. Before a pregnancy is terminated, the women must be informed of the significance and effects of the operation. She must then be given advice on contraception. The above conditions also apply to minors. There are no legal regulations covering the advertisement of abortion.	Implementation of this law is regarded as highly effective and illegal abortion is rare. State hospital provision for abortion is supplemented by a private clinic sector.
7. Infertility treatment	This subject is not covered by law.	Infertility treatment is available from hospitals free of charge, and Väestöliitto, the Finnish FPA.
8. Sex education/family life education	Sex education/family life education is included in the school curricula by Government provision at all levels of teaching from nursery school to higher education.	Sex education, where provided, is spread throughout a range of subjects: civics, biology, home economics etc. The content however, is dependent upon the individual school. It is believed that the legal provision for sex education in schools is reflected in practice, particularly in the lowest levels of educational provisions (nursery). Actual provision at the higher levels does not so well reflect the legal directives.

Issue	De Jure	De Facto
9. Adoption	The adoption law came into effect in 1980. Adopted children have equal status in law as other children. Respectively, the juridical relation of the adopted child to his/her natural parents will be totally severed. Adoption counselling is compulsory for those wishing to adopt. A child over 11 years is permitted to give his/her own written consent regarding the adoption.	No data.

Issue	De Jure	De Facto
1. Government recognition of human right to number and spacing of children (planned parenthood)	No Government recognition of the right.	Legislation of 1974 involved the State in the provision of free contraception, giving some recognition to the right of an individual to family planning. There is no legal age restriction on access to contraception. Contraceptives are paid for by the client and the cost reimbursed, all or in part, through the social security system (except barrier and spermicide methods).
Protection of family and child	Protection of family and child is enshrined in the Constitution (2 November 1945), and indirectly in the public health code of 1962.	These State services exist as separate clinics (Protection maternelle et Infantile, PMI); as part of hospitals PMI clinics; and in other centres such as municiple health centres. However, in general these centres do not offer specialised services for specific groups (e.g. women only, adolescents only). However, there are also non-Government (private) centres for fp help: MFPF centres; MGEN centres (enseignants); UDMT (travailleurs).
2. Government and other family planning (fp) facilities/services	A range of laws govern the State family planning services. The provision of advice on contraception is encouraged by these laws.	In general, family planning centres are poorly distributed in France, certain regions being particularly deprived. In some cases there is only one centre per department. The rural and mountainous regions are very poorly served. Moreover, the hours of opening of the centres are often arranged to suit the woman staying at home (during school hours) and therefore do not accommodate the needs of young and/or working women. In recent years, partly through the initiative of centre personnel and partly through the initiative of the MFPF, opening hours have become more flexible (e.g. the opening hours on Wednesday afternoons for young people). Contraceptives are also supplied by liberal GPs, other physicians and gynaecologists.
3. The sale, distribution and advertisement of contraceptives	There is no legal impediment to the sale of contraceptives. The sale of contraceptives in pharmacies is permitted where authorisation has been received by the Ministry of Social Affairs. Distribution of contraceptives from fp or family education centres is not permitted with exception of the provision for minors requesting anonymity.	Since 1980, the addresses of fp centres were supposed to be on display in certain public places: hospitals, pharmacies etc. Very often this was not the case. Since 1981, all fp addresses have been published by the Government, and they can be found in town halls and post offices.

Issue	De Jure	De Facto
	Pharmacies supply IUDs on medical prescription. A physician's prescription is required for oral contraceptives and IUDs. A decree of 7th March 1972 and a statutory instrument of 2nd Apr. 1982 prescribe the conditions under which IUDs may be inserted by physicians only. There are no special regulations regarding condoms and diaphragms. Appliance methods are sold without restriction in pharmacies only - except condoms, which can be purchased in a few of the large stores.	No publicity is provided for contraception per se, though it is provided through the information which identifies the location of services for the public. In spite of circular 4.185, much remains to be done, as few centres are effectively advertised.
	All propaganda and commercial advertising of contraceptives in the mass media is forbidden by law. Advertising in the medical press is only permitted on a special Ministry of Social Affairs permit.	
4. Availability/sale of family planning (fp) related literature.	Circular 4.185 of 16th March 1983 of the Ministry of Health decrees that widespread publication for fp centres should be given through posters, advertisements etc. of opening times and services. There is nothing in the law which forbids the sale/dissemination of fp related literature.	A small amount of literature is available, sometimes through libraries, bookshops and MFPF centres, and Women's/young people's magazines: eg. 'OK' magazine which is an important source of fairly accurate information. Some associations convey a contraceptive message in accordance with their objectives. Thus, the Ministry of Women's Rights, concerned with the lack of available leaflets for the general public, has produced a leaflet, 'Contraception: A Basic Right', distributed free-of-charge.
5. Sterilisation	There are no laws governing sterilisation per se. However, sterilisation could in theory be legally challenged by invoking a decree which forbids mutilation of the body for reasons other than disease.	In practice, physicians perform some thousands of vasectomies and many more female sterilisations each year, for fp purposes. Such physicians may demand to know the age/number of existing children of those requesting sterilisation and, where appropriate, the written consent of the husband, though this has no legal status.

Issue	De Jure	De Facto
	As sterilisation as a fp method has no status under law, it is not recognised by the social security code and therefore cannot be reimbursed through this system.	In fact most are reimbursed in a rather hypocritical way.
6. Abortion	Induced abortion is legally regulated by law No. 75/17 1975. Abortion on request is authorised up to the 10th week of pregnancy for a woman who is deemed to be in a 'state of distress'. There are restrictions for minors and foreigners. A physician approached with a request for abortion must inform the women of the medical risks to herself and any future pregnancy; provide in writing details of State entitlements, family benefits/allowances, adoption possibilities (should she decide to continue with the pregnancy); and a list of organisations which she could turn to for assistance. Women desiring abortion must obtain, from appropriate/recognised institutions (e.g. fp centres) a certificate of referral for consultation which describes the nature and purpose of counselling, and recommends attendance by both partners. If a woman, after such counselling, wishes to proceed, the physician must receive written confirmation which may only become effective one week after the first request is made. Having received confirmation, the physician may perform an abortion according to the following conditions: an abortion may only be performed by a physician in a public hospital or registered private clinic satisfying certain criteria; the number of abortions may not exceed one quarter of the total number of operations performed in any one establishment; health personnel have the right to refuse to participate in an abortion for reasons of conscience. In the last case, the physician refers the woman to another physician or one of her choice, together with a certificate to the effect that the conditions above have been fulfilled. That is, a physician is not obliged to process a request for or perform an abortion, but must inform the client of his/her refusal to do so.	Past governments have not effectively implemented the right to legal abortion. The present government is considering revising the conditions to facilitate access to abortion. In autumn 1983, in certain regions it remained difficult for a woman to find an outlet for abortion. While the situation varies from one city to another, in general there are not enough hospital beds. About 40% of abortions are performed in clinics, and the situation worsens in the Summer, since abortion is not considered a matter of urgency and physicians are often not replaced. Certain abortion centres in hospitals are closed for one or two months.

Issue	De Jure	De Facto
6. Abortion (contd.)	The cost of the abortion and of hospitalisation is determined by the public authority, and since 1983 a woman is reimbursed 80% of the cost. Therapeutic abortion may be performed where two experts recognised by tribunal agree, after consultation, that the continuation of a pregnancy would represent a grave danger to the health of the woman or where there is a strong likelihood that the child would suffer from grave defects. Abortion is not legally regarded as a method of contraception.	Hospitals are obliged to apply these price rates. The clinics often apply the rates they wish to, and physicians, particularly in the clinics, often charge more than the prescribed rate. Furthermore, in principle, women are supposed to benefit from the so-called 'one-third payment', as for other medical interventions. That is, she is only supposed to pay the remainder in the case of abortion: 20% of the charge. It is extremely difficult to ensure that all the clinics do this, but most of the clinics refuse, obliging the woman to advance the full sum and only thereafter is she able to obtain a reimbursement from social security.
7. Infertility	Although recognised as a treatment for infertility, artificial insemination (AI) may be performed without legal codification. In 1980, a senator (M. Caillavet) proposed a text which is in the process of adoption by the Senate. AI may only be performed by a physician upon the written request of both spouses. There is no remuneration for sperm donation. The treatment/conservation of the donor sperm must be conducted by an officially recognised organisation. There AI may be possible only for married women. These regulations have yet to be sanctioned by the National Assembly.	In practice, it is difficult for even married couples to obtain AI; more difficult still for non-married couples and lesbians.
8. Sex education/family life education	Information on sexual matters is included in the schedule curriculum by Government provision. Since 1973 an official notice regulates separately sex information and sex education. The responsibility for sex information was given to schools, to be included within the curriculum of natural sciences. It was permitted that meetings on this subject could be held after school hours.	In practice, the 1973 legislation has only been partially recognised and implemented by schools. Texts have been produced to fulfill the needs of teachers and science textbooks have been modified to include such information. There is, however, no standardisation and the majority of texts do not deal with contraception satisfactorily.

Issue	De Jure	De Facto
8. Sex Education/family life education (contd).	In the first level (up to 14-15 years) students may be admitted to sex information classes upon a written authorisation from their parents. In the second level they may be freely admitted to such classes without prior authorisation from parents (though parents can withhold their children from such classes if they declare their objections in a written note). Teachers will generally not partake in these classes, which are conducted, rather, by specialists in the field brought in from outside the school who have received the training authorised by the law. The parents of the students must have the opportunity to sanction the organisation invited to the school. Officially, sex education was deemed the responsibility of parents. Since December 1981, according to a circular, sex education is officially the responsibility of the Ministry of National Education, and teachers and all teaching staff should be trained in this.	No budget was allocated by the Ministry of Education to ensure the implementation of the 1973 legislation. Hence the field remains dominated by competing organisations – from Catholic groups to the Movement Francais pour le Planning Familial. Morale both among teachers and students is low concerning the quality and potential of the subject in the school setting. In general, the legislation is not reflected in practice at all at nursery school level; a small amount in elementary schools; there is 'theoretical' implementation in all secondary schools; and the subject is non-existent in higher education establishments. In sum, the content of sex information is dependent upon the attitudes of the schools, i.e. the personnel therein. There is a little sex education provided in the youth club setting and MFPF centres have organised youth discussion groups for many years. Very little attention is given to the subject by the mass media. Thus, legal provision for sex information/education is not reflected in practice. At the beginning of 1984 numerous Lycee students, having completed their final secondary studies, report receiving no sex education in the schools. Numerous training courses have been organised by head teachers through different organisations, including the MFPF. However, there are financial problems in organising courses and needs remain unmet.
9. Adoption	In order to qualify for adoption the couple must have been married five years with one of the partners over 35 years, the couple applying jointly. Adoption is open to anyone over 35 years. The adoptee's consent is required over 15 years old.	There is a lack of French children for adoption.

Issue	De Jure	De Facto
1. Government recognition of human right to number and spacing of children (planned parenthood)	Government recognition is not legally or otherwise specified.	In practice the Government supports fp facilities and services. There is close cooperation between the board of the GDR FPA and the Ministry of Health. For example, the recommendation of the GDR FPA was taken into consideration in the Government decision to legalise abortion in 1972.
Protection of family and child	The Constitution explicitly states that marriage and the family enjoy the protection of the State. Single parent- and large families are given special assistance. Mother and child receive the benefits of pregnancy leave and child receive the benefits of pregnancy leave and child allowance.	
	The Family Law includes a paragraph (4) by which the administration of centres of population must establish counselling centres (1966). In 1968, the Ministry of Health issued guidelines covering medical personnel in these centres, including family planning as a main task.	In principle, the Government practices a pronatalist policy. However, this is not reflected in any restriction on the practice of contraception or abortion.
2. Government and other family planning (fp) facilities/services	Legislation on family planning facilities exists only relating to female sterilisation.	In practice, the Government supports fp facilities, most of them integrated into the national health service. Such services are offered through hospitals, general practitioners, gynaecologists and family planning centres and are generally free-of-charge. There are no private or specialised fp centres. Family planning services are often integrated with counselling services, which deal with psychosexual and marital problems for both sexes. In some towns, special services for adolescents have been established.
		There are around 200 centres in the GDR through which fp services are offered situated to cover rural as well as urban areas. Urban centres are better attended - even by rural dwellers who prefer to escape from the familiarity of their own locale. Adolescent services are also well attended.
3. The sale, distribution and advertisement of contraceptives	The sale/distribution of contraceptives is not forbidden by law. However, they are legally regulated.	There is no general advertising of contraceptives, though magazine/newspaper articles do feature contraceptive method issues. Similarly, television will refer to fp centres when features on contraception are produced.
		A woman obtains the pill from a pharmacy, through the prescription received from a physician. IUDs are obtained through

Issue	De Jure	De Facto
	There is no law covering the advertisement of contraceptives.	gynaecological departments of clinics/hospitals. Condoms are available through pharmacies, vending machines and mail order (via newspaper advertisements). Condoms alone must be paid for, and no legal limitations exist on their sale. Although available in some clinics, the diaphragm is unpopular and rarely used. With the exception of condoms, no contraceptives are advertised.
4. Availability/sale of family planning (fp) related literature.	No law forbids the sale or distribution of fp related literature.	This literature is readily available from bookshops and libraries.
		A special booklet aimed at young people was edited in 1983 and will be used in schools. Over the last 10 years, a number of books on sex education, sexual problems and contraception have been produced - mostly by members of the FPA. One was specially designed for teachers, another for young children (3-6 years). The demand is great for this material.
5. Sterilisation	Sterilisation is legally permitted as a method of contraception as well as for medical reasons for women only. A law is in preparation to cover the male.	Male sterilisation is available only for medical reasons. Sterilisation for women is available on request, though a 'commission of experts' decides if it should be performed or not. In most cases, sterilisations are performed because women are unable to take the pill or use an IUD because of unacceptable side-effects, and already have completed their families. Sterilisation is officially called 'irreversible contraception'.
6. Abortion	Since 1972, abortion has been legal, permitted on request up to the 12th week of pregnancy. After this time it is permitted principally on medical grounds only, with the consent of a committee of medical and social authorities. The performing physician is obliged to inform the woman of possible side-effects of the operation and to provide contraceptive advice. Minors must have the consent of their parents.	In practice, abortion is readily available, requiring that a woman simply approach her GP. There is no evidence of any large-scale illegal abortion. No private abortion clinics exist, and all treatment is carried out in national health service hospitals.

Issue	De Jure	De Facto
7. Infertility treatment	No legal regulations govern infertility treatment or artificial insemination.	The family planning service does not regard infertility treatment as part of the services it is responsible for. However, counselling on the subject is undertaken for the purposes of referral. Clients with infertility problems are referred to special medical departments, andrological as well as gynaecological, where psychological as well as physical tests can be carried out. AID is available through special centres, following the written agreement of the couple that any child will be regarded as legitimate.
8. Sex education/family life education	Sex education/family life education is included in the school curriculum by Government provision. Though not specified by law, the content is dictated by regulations covering other parts of the curriculum.	Although it is believed that the legal directives on sex education are covered in practice, the quality of this education differs widely by school and region, and according to the commitment of the teachers concerned.
9. Adoption	Adoption is regulated by legislation concerning the family. An adopted child shall have a home suitable to the good upbringing of the child. Adopter and adoptee are legally bound by the same regulations covering natural-born children.	In general, there is a shortage of adoptees, as availability of abortion has removed the possibility of unwanted births. The Referat Jugendhilfe is responsible for adoption arrangements including assessment of the suitability of the potential adopters. At present there is a waiting time for a child of between 1 and 2 years. Consent of the child's parents to an adoption is necessary (as well as that of the child itself) if the child is over 14 years old.

Issue	De Jure	De Facto
1. Government recognition of human right to number and spacing of children (planned parenthood)	The right of an individual to free determination of the number and spacing of children is not regulated by law.	It is believed that nevertheless such rights are respected by Government in practice. Family planning services are incorporated within the national health system.
Protection of family and child	Protection of family and child is written into the Constitution as follows: 'The Hungarian People's Republic protects the institution of marriage and family. The Hungarian People's Republic pays special attention to the development and social education of young people and protects their interests'.	
2. Government and other family planning (fp) facilities/services	There is no law strictly covering the subject of family planning, though decrees do exist relating to certain methods of fertility regulation, viz: abortion, oral and intra-uterine contraception. No law covers the advertisement of fp clinics.	State family planning services exist as part of hospital and Mother & Child Health care centres and offer specialised services for women only. Sexual counselling is also available. No private fp facilities exist. In rural areas family planning is the task of the district physician, within the activity of welfare of mothers and children, and in strict cooperation with the district nurses. They may rely on counselling service of the Regional hospital out-patients clinic. Contraceptives are subsidised by the State.
		The Ministry of Health provides for the training of all physicians working in the above fields. All physicians performing the family planning service may prescribe oral contraceptives, but IUDs may be inserted only in hospitals, thus the gynaecological departments of the hospitals decide on this matter. Post coital contraception is available on prescription.
		The tasks of the Counselling Units for Family and Women's Welfare are as follows: counselling concerning contracaption; prenatal care; treatment of infertility; treatments after an unsuccessful pregnancy; gynaecological treatments for children; oncological screening tests; premarital counselling; genetical counselling; andrological counselling; psychological counselling; legal counselling. The last four services are not provided by all the counselling units for Family and Women's Welfare, only by some selected units.

- 89 -

Issue	De Jure	De Facto
		Counselling units exist in all hospitals in the country. In areas without hospitals it is undertaken by physicians, or in their absence the factory doctor. Advertising of the service is unnecessary as this is incorporated within publicity relating to general public health.
3. The sale, distribution and advertisement of contraception.	There is no law dealing explicitly with the advertisement of contraceptives. No law forbids the sale of contraceptives.	Contraceptives can be purchased mainly in pharmacies; orals may be obtained only through medical prescription. IUD's are issued only on the basis of a medical prescription and they may be inserted only in hospitals where surgical intervention is available for treatment of possible complications. Spermicides and condoms may be purchased in pharmacies. Condoms can also be bought in perfumeries and household stores. The price of all contraceptives is very low.
4. Availability/sale of family planning (fp) related literature.	No law forbids the sale of fp related literature.	Contraceptives are not advertised as most are obtained through the national health service. Books, booklets and leaflets on family planning are produced by the health service. They can be purchased from medical waiting rooms, bookshops, street, booksellers. Information is also available through magazines.
5. Sterilisation		The health law permits operations only for the protection of health, so legally it is not possible to carry out sterilisation as contraception. In practice in some cases women may be sterilised in a secondary operation if through this further impairing of health is prevented. For example, after two cesarean sections the operation may be carried out on request. The Hungarian Scientific Society for Family and Women's Welfare prepared a draft concerning the authorization of voluntary sterilization operations for contraception for the Health Ministry.

Issue	De Jure	De Facto
6. Abortion	Interruption of pregnancy is authorised within the first 12 weeks, on request, by a committee established for this purpose. The committee authorises an abortion if: the woman is single; the woman is 35+; she is unsuitably housed; she already has 3 children, or if she has 2 children and medical complications; she is suffering from ill-health, or bad social conditions. In general, women have to pay for the operation, though her financial status is taken into consideration. The highest charge is about $22. For minors the consent of a legal representative is necessary.	Legal abortion is available through the state health system.
7. Infertility treatment	Artificial insemination is regulated by law: 'Insemination by means of an operation might be carried out on request on a woman under 40 years old, married, and a Hungarian Citizen, where according to medical opinion there is a great probability that no healthy child could be born of her marriage naturally'. The law also regulates the application procedure for artificial insemination, the circumstances of the carrying out of the operation, and the legal status of the child born in such a way.	No data.
8. Sex education/family life education	Education for family life is included in schools at primary, secondary and third levels. The content has been developed centrally. Such education is also provided in the army.	Sex education is carried out in schools and in the army. In schools pupils receive sex education in biology lessons. Teachers acquire the knowledge necessary for teaching family life education in courses designed for this purpose. However, as yet, family life education is not a mandatory subject within all teacher training colleges and universities.
9. Adoption	A part of the Family Law deals with adoption: 'The purpose of adoption is to establish a family relation between the adoptant, as well as his/her relatives, and the adoptee; and most importantly, to ensure a family education for minors who have no parents or who cannot be educated properly by their parents'.	The conditions of adoption are regulated by the family law. Children for adoption are in great demand. The authorities permitting the adoption take into consideration the interest of the adoptee and therefore they have certain requirements in respect of couples desiring to adopt children. The authorities examine to what extent the conditions of the couple will ensure the undisturbed education and the balanced emotional development of the child.

Issue	De Jure	De Facto
1. Government recognition of human right to the number and spacing of children (planned parenthood).	The right of the individual to decide on the number and spacing of children is specified in the Health (Family Planning) Act 1979 and - in Government regulations pertaining to it and a 1985 amendment. The Government is also a signatory of the Teheran Proclamation 1968.	In practice this right is vaguely specified in the Health (Family Planning) Act. It discriminates against providing this right to certain social groups because the State only provides finance for 'natural' family planning (fp) methods (where fp is prescribed for medical reasons). Restrictions in the Health (Family Planning) Act on the sale and distribution of medical contraceptives also denies people this right (see below).
Protection of family and child.	The protection of illegitimate children is not afforded under the Constitution.	Illegitimate children are discriminated against within the present legal system. At present, illegitimate children have no succession rights, though this law may be amended in the near future. Also, they have less access to welfare benefits, qualifying the mother for an unmarried mother's allowance rather than the full family allowance.
2. Government and other family planning (fp) services/facilities	Fp facilities have been regulated within the 1979 Act. This Act made provision for fp services, with a view to ensuring that contraceptives are available for 'bona fide' family planning purposes only. The spirit of the law here was to restrict access to married couples only. Only a registered medical practitioner was authorised to provide prescriptions for contraceptives to be obtained only from a pharmacist.

A 1985 Amendment to the Act liberalised the manner and means of distribution of 'non-medical contraceptives' (condoms/spermicides), making them available to any person over 18 years without prescription/without consultation with a physician/pharmacist. | Under the conditions of the 1979 Act, the Health Boards (local health authorities) were compelled to provide natural family planning methods only, provided through hospitals/Mother & Child Health care (MCH) clinics. However, see De Jure. Some antenatal clinics do distribute literature on the other methods.

There are at least 9 non-Government family planning clinics in Ireland which offer most methods for payment and subsist only on income received.

Only a limited number of pharmacists offer this service. Most private fp clinics advertise their services. |
| 3. The sale, distribution and advertisement of contraceptives | Distribution/sale of contraceptives are regulated by the Pharmacy Acts 1895-1977, as well as the Health (Family Planning) Act 1979. The 1985 Amendment permits distribution/sale of condoms/spermicides through fp clinics health boards, hospitals, sexually transmitted disease services, pharmacies, and GPs.

Contraceptive advertising is illegal. | Contraceptives are sold in private fp clinics, in some student union centres, and by GPs. |

Issue	De Jure	De Facto
4. Availability/sale of fp related literature.	Consumer fp literature is not readily available though it can be obtained from the private (IFPA) clinic network. The State issues no literature.	British women's magazines, which regularly feature family planning issues, are widely available/read in Ireland.
5. Sterilisation	Sterilisation is not legally regulated as fp within the 1979 Act, and is therefore technically available to those wishing to resort to it as an fp method.	In practice, female sterilisation requires (State) hospitalisation. However, State hospital 'ethical' committees generally refuse permission for the operation to be performed. One Health Board recently formally announced that no requests for sterilisation would be considered in its area. Moreover, the majority of nurses would refuse to partake in such operations because of religious persuasion. However, female sterilisation is available in two private hospitals in Ireland, though this is expensive and waiting lists are long. As a result women are usually referred to England. Vasectomies are performed in a few private fp clinics on an outpatient basis.
6. Abortion	Abortion is legally forbidden without exception under the 1861 Offences Against the Person Act. The right to life of the unborn foetus is now protected under the 8th Amendment of the Irish Constitution (1983).	There is an abortion referral service (to England) in Dublin run by the 'Open Door' Counselling Service. It is estimated that 5,000 women per year use the service—estimated to be about 50% of those who actually obtain abortions. All private fp clinics offer pregnancy counselling and post-abortion check-ups.
7. Infertility treatment	Infertility treatment is not legally regulated.	In practice, there are only very few specialists working in this field. Two private fp clinics offer infertility referral services.
8. Sex education/family life education	Sex education is not included in the school curriculum by Government provision. The Department of Education believes that responsibility for such education rests with parents. Individual schools are permitted to provide such education if they so choose.	In practice, sex education does not appear in the school curriculum, though such education is offered by some nurses, teachers, probation officers, and youth workers. The Health Education Bureau has begun to draw up a programme for second level schools.

Issue	De Jure	De Facto
		The IFPA provides resources and training courses for professionals working with young people in this field.
9. Adoption	Adoption of children is regulated under the law (Adoption Acts 1952-1976). A couple is entitled to adopt a child provided they are over 25 and have been married a minimum of 3 years. The adoptee must be a resident of Ireland, between the ages of 6 months and 7 years, and illegitimate or orphaned.	No data.

Issue	De Jure	De Facto
1. Government recognition of human right to number and spacing of children. (planned parenthood)	This is specified in Law No. 405 of July, 1975 and is reiterated in the Abortion Act of 1978 which, in recognising the social value of motherhood provides for the State's guarantee of the right to conscious and responsible procreation and the protection of human life from its inception. (Art.1). It also provides (Art.2) that under-age people shall also have access in the health services and in the family planning clinics, and on medical prescription, to the means necessary for freely-chosen and responsible procreation.	In practice, planned parenthood as a human right is not completely respected. Although legal regulation of family planning facilities and services, contraceptive sale and distribution, and abortion is generally protective and enabling, full implementation of the law is undermined by lack of services and facilities for rural and under-privileged groups, particularly in the south. There is anabsence of contraceptive information, and an extraordinarily high rate of conscientious objection on moral and religious grounds declared by members of the medical and health professions.
Protection of the family and child	This is constitutionally guaranteed and supported directly by special family laws and indirectly by other laws and regulations: e.g. Abortion Act; Mother and Child Health Care Act.	
2. Government and other family planning (fp) facilities/services	Family planning clinics and associated services, both public and voluntary, were legally established and are legally regulated by Law No. 405 of July 1975 and by the Abortion Act (Law No. 194) of May 1978. The 1975 law provides for free family planning services.	In 1981 the Minister of Health declared that there were about 1,200 public family planning clinics throughout Italy. They are, however, most heavily concentrated in the north and central regions and available information indicates that facilities and services are still virtually non-existent in the Islands and southern regions of Italy. Both government (separate clinics) and non-government (private) fp facilities and services are available. The Government offers both health services (contraception, preventive medicine) and psychosocial services (information, counselling therapy) to men, women, couples, and adolescents. However, facilities and services are inadequate or virtually non-existent in some areas, particulary in the south.

Issue	De Jure	De Facto
3. The sale, distribution and advertisement of contraceptives.	No legal prohibition exists against the manufacture, import or sale of contraceptives, although distribution of medical contraceptives (pills and IUD) are legally regulated. They can be obtained only through pharmacies on a prescription basis. All other contraceptives are available from pharmacies, and vending machines, etc. The law states that medical contraceptives may be advertised only in professional literature and magazines for scientific information purposes. By law, non-medical contraceptives may be freely advertised.	Contraceptives are available free of charge in the public sector and can be purchased in the private sector.
4. Availability/sale of family planning (fp) related literature.	The production and sale of consumer literature related to fp is not forbidden by law.	Production and availability of consumer literature is generally limited to that produced and distributed by FP clinics or other local health services.
5. Sterilisation	There is no law governing sterilisation as such, though the legality of the method could theoretically be challenged according to a law which prohibits mutilation of the body.	In the absence of a law, there is at present confusion over the government position – as a result very few public hospitals offer the service. However, where available it is free-of-charge. Some private fp centres are active in this field, providing sterilisation for payment.
6. Abortion	Induced abortion is legally regulated. The Abortion Act adopted in 1978 was endorsed by a referendum in May 1981. Under the Act abortion is permitted on medical and socio-economic grounds up to 12 weeks of pregnancy. The Act applies to minors (under 16 years) provided consent is obtained from parents or a judge. There is no law which specifically prohibits the advertisement of abortion.	Legal provisions on abortion are not altogether effective or fully implemented due to the fact that only a few private clinics have sought or obtained the required authorisation and there is considerable conscientious objection on religious, moral and social grounds. In practice, advertisement of abortion is non-existent. Illegal abortions are still numerous, practiced on a large scale, though the 1978 legislation and 1981 referendum are expected to reduce this practice.

Issue	De Jure	De Facto
	Legally abortions may be performed in hospitals and private clinics authorised by the regional authorities. Women requesting abortions within the time limit must obtain a doctor's certificate and wait for a minimum of 7 days.	The law is more fully implemented in the North and central Regions than in the South, where facilities and services are lacking in both the public and private sector. Due to shortage of private clinics, most abortions are now carried out in hospitals where they are provided free-of-charge.
7. Infertility treatment	Infertility treatment and AID are not legally regulated.	No data
8. Sex education/family life education	There is no legal or Government provision for including sex education/family life education in school curricula. By law, sex education can be provided in schools with the consent of parents.	Sex education is available in some schools, though the content varies according to the prevailing attitudes. Sex education is also to some extent treated in the mass media.
9. Adoption	Adoption is legally regulated. The adopter must be more than 35 years old, and at least 18 years older than the proposed adoptee. In exceptional circumstances a court may authorise adoption where the adopter is over 30 years old. It is possible to adopt only if one has no existing legitimate or illegitimate children. If the adoptee is over 12 years old then his/her consent is required.	No data.

- 97 -

Issue	De Jure	De Facto
1. Government recognition of human right to number and spacing of children (planned parenthood)	The rights of the individual to free choice in the number and spacing of children is taken as legally specified due to national commitment to an international convention for the protection of human rights and fundamental freedoms. Article 12 of the Constitution states that: 'Men and women of marriageable age have the right to marry and found a family according to the national laws governing the exercise of this right'.	Government recognition of this right, de facto, has recently been reaffirmed through renewed financial support for the Rutgers Stichting, the Dutch FPA.
2. Government and other family planning (fp) facilities/services	Family planning services are legally regulated. The law allows for certain kinds of advertisement of fp clinics.	There are no government family planning facilities; all services are private, fee-paying. Some private fp services are subsidised by the government. There are 40 Rutgers Stichting (RS) sex counselling/family planning centres (fee-paying FPA network) which are preferred to local GP fp services by many (mainly middle class) women. Nevertheless, the majority of women in the Netherlands will utilise GPs for their family planning needs. There is very good cooperation between GPs and the RS centres, to which many women/young people are referred for more specialised help (counselling etc.). The younger generation of GPs are being trained in family planning to a greater degree than the older generation and are likely to be more popular with the public in the future. Nevertheless, at present, more than 50% of GPs feel less than competent to provide sexual/fp counselling; and 20% feel unhappy about providing oral contraceptives to teenagers in the 15-18 age group on moral grounds. The RS centres are advertised occasionally in newspapers, and a recent RS book is now available to the public through 6000 selling outlets.
3. The sale, distribution and advertisement of contraceptives	The sale of contraceptives is not legally forbidden. The distribution of contraceptives is legally regulated according to manufacturing standards.	Around 50% of oral contraceptors are members of health insurance schemes which reimburse the cost of pills. The remainder pay the full price.

- 98 -

Issue	De Jure	De Facto
	Condoms can be bought anywhere: from shops, automatic vending machines and so on. Oral contraceptives are available from pharmacies only through prescription from a physician. The cost of oral contraceptives can be reimbursed through health insurance	Oral contraceptives cost the public around $1 per pack. Condoms are also inexpensive and available in numerous outlets. Nevertheless, the cost of contraceptives could still inhibit use particularly by the unemployed young. In principle, every GP is supposed to be able to insert an IUD. However, many do not feel themselves skillful enough and refer patients to gynaecologists/RS. Many women prefer to pay for insertion by Rutgers Stichting professionals (20,000 in 1982). There are around 100,000 IUD users in the Netherlands, 50% of whom utilised RS centres. There exists some free 'public advertising' on Netherlands TV which has been used in the past to provide warning about STDs. Condoms have been, on occasion, advertised commercially.
4. Availability/sale of family planning (fp) related literature	No law forbids the dissemination of fp-related literature.	Consumer literature is readily available from fp clinics, bookshops, public libraries, RS counselling bureaux, youth centres. Most GPs have literature to provide free to the public on request.
5. Sterilisation	There is no law governing sterilisation, though it is available as a family planning method for both men and women. The operation is 'free' insofar as its cost is reimbursed through health insurance schemes, whether State or private, if performed in officially-recognised licensed institutions.	There have been up to 100,000 sterilisations per annum (50%-50% sex ratio) though the number has declined to around 50,000 in 1982. There are adequate services to meet demand. Sterilisations are paid for either through the State or private insurance schemes, and operations are performed in hospitals on an out-patient basis. Sterilisation is performed in abortion clinics free-of-charge.

Issue	De Jure	De Facto
6. Abortion	A Bill was passed permitting legal abortion in 1981; administrative regulations were finalised in 1984.	In the absence of a fully operating Abortion Law, hospitals and clinics conduct between them (in ratio of 1:3) around 20,000 abortions p.a.
	The new law introduces certain restrictive conditions:	It is believed that there is no evidence that illegal abortion is performed on a large scale.
	1.The consent of a physician with a 5 day compulsory 'conscience' period between referral and actual service in clinic or hospital. 2.Restrictions on the clinics that perform abortions to limit access. 3.The requirement that after the 13th week, further requirements are to be fulfilled for the clinics.	Abortion clinics are in fact dependent on the willingness of a neighbouring hospital to make a contract to cooperate with the clinic on the board level in order to receive a licence from the Ministry of Health to perform abortions.
	It is likely that legalisation of abortion will end the necessity of payment (₤100) The operation will not be subject to reimbursement through existing health insurance schemes.	
7. Infertility	There are no legal regulations covering infertility treatment.	Everyone who needs infertility services can obtain all necessary tests free of charge within the health system.
8. Sex education/family life education	Sex education is not included in the school curriculum by Govt. provision. However, a law has been drafted to achieve this and is awaiting approval.	Sex education is available at all levels of education though its quantity and quality is unmonitored and dependent upon the school concerned. It is likely that a new sex education law will be approved in 1985 (Health education with a sex education component). At present many schools request Rutgers Stichting teachers to come into schools to provide instruction, though this will depend upon the decisions of the school head. A recent survey of young people reported that 30% stated that they had received most of their sexual knowledge from the school. As the State does not provide this component of education, there is great demand for RS services.
		It is also available through youth clubs, evening classes for adults and is covered by the mass media.

Issue	De Jure	De Facto
9. Adoption	Adoption is legally regulated. The adopter must be at least 18 years older than the adoptee, and at the most 50 years older. If the child is 12 years or older its consent is also necessary. The adoptee should be younger than 16. It is legally difficult to adopt a person older than 16.	The demand for Dutch children exceeds supply (though such children of 8 years and older are more available for adoption). This vacuum has been filled by the 'legal' and illegal buying of children from the Third World.

Issue	De Jure	De Facto
1. Government recognition of human right to number and spacing of children (planned parenthood)	The Norwegian Government has committed itself to international declarations and conventions which include such recognition.	Largely, Mother and Child Health care (MCH) clinics have provided family planning services, though these have been augmented by non-governmental social welfare organisations where Government services were not available. However, from 1984, every community will have a family planning clinic funded by the State and community.
Protection of family and child	This issue is covered by a special family law. From the beginning of 1984, this subject will be covered by a new health services law. The Penal Code of 1902 forbids intercourse with a girl under 16 years.	
2. Government and other family planning (fp) facilities/services	Legislation on fp facilities exists in the context of the Mother and Child Health care law and the Abortion law. No law forbids the advertising of clinics.	Family planning clinics are provided by Government, as separate clinics and as part of hospitals, MCH centres. These offer special services for both sexes independently, and for adolescents andmigrants seperately. Psychosexual counselling is also available. Private clinics also exist (10-15 centres).
3. The sale, distribution and advertisement of contraceptives	There are no legal regulations forbidding the sale of contraceptives. With the exception of oral contraceptives which must be obtained by prescription in pharmacies, there are no legal regulations covering the distribution of contraceptives. No law forbids contraceptive advertising, though oral contraceptive advertising requires Ministry of Health approval.	Contraceptives are not free of charge though inexpensive. Non-prescriptive contraceptives can be obtained in petrol stations, ordinary shops, most pharmacies and by mail order.
4. Availability/sale of fp related literature	There are no legal regulations forbidding the availability/sale of fp related literature.	This material is readily available from clinics, libraries (including school libraries), bookshops, and the Norwegian FPA.
5. Sterilisation	Sterilisation is legally regulated and is permitted as a fp method for men and women. It is provided on request to those over 25 years old.	The law is reflected in practice. Both male and female sterilisations have increased, and presently run at circa 6000 per annum.
6. Abortion	Abortion is legally permitted on request up to the 12th week of pregnancy. It is permitted after the 12th week on application.	It is believed that State and community family counselling services cover the needs of the population.

Issue	De Jure	De Facto
6. Abortion (contd).	Abortion and community services are provided by the State health services free of charge. Private abortion services do not exist. The advertisement of abortion services is legally regulated.	
7. Infertility treatment	There are no legal regulations covering infertility treatment. It is regarded as the affair of the doctor and patient.	In Oslo and Trondheim there exist special infertility services as part of the general health services. Treatment is provided through hospitals, though the demand for this service is greater than can be provided for.
8. Sex education/family life education	Sex education is included in the school curriculum by Government provision.	In practice it is only partly implemented in the secondary school level alone, and to some extent in youth clubs. TV and radio also deal with the subject to some extent. The content is dependent upon the school itself and only crudely covered in terms of legal directives.

With the exception of basic biological information, sex education training is not included in the teacher training curriculum. The regulations state, however, that family planning should be part of the school curriculum from 1st to 9th grade (16 years), appropriate to the child's understanding.

Sex education issues often appear in magazines and newspapers, and more seldomly on radio, and very rarely on TV. Public opinion concerning sex education for young people is liberal, though there are objections to the provision of contraceptive information to girls under 16 years old, without parental consent. |
| 9. Adoption | The law states that a man or woman 25 years or over may adopt a child. Children over 12 years cannot be adopted without their own consent. It is forbidden for private persons to arrange adoptions, which must be supervised by the Health Service Office of the community, or a children's consultant in the district who is responsible for this subject. | Adoption is rare in Norway due mainly to the strong economic situation of young mothers. However, there are many Norwegian couples who wish to adopt foreign children, and the Social Department has regulations covering the acceptability of potential adopters. |

Issue	De Jure	De Facto
1. Government recognition of human right to number and spacing of children (planned parenthood)	The right of the individual to free determination of the number and spacing of children is not legally regulated in the form of a specific law.	In practice, specific laws and regulations (on abortion, contraception, child-care) secure this right, or at least create no legal barriers. Particularly during 1976-83, many special provisions in favour of large families and young working mothers were initiated (eg maternity-leave up to 3 years with partial pay and job guarantee).
Protection of family and child	Protection of the family and child is noted in the Constitution, 1976, which explicitly states that families with many children should receive special State assistance.	
2. Government and other family planning (fp) facilities/services	Family planning facilities/services are registered. Only physicians specialised in gynaecology and specially trained nurses may insert IUDs (Ministry of Health and Social Welfare, 1 April 1963). Official distribution is concentrated in the Public Health Service under Regulation 34 of 1960.	The public is served by Government fp clinics, usually part of hospitals or Mother and Child Health (MCH) centres. The Polish PPA offers 15 private clinics and up to 20 marital counselling centres (some shared with the State). There are many Roman Catholic counselling centres. No fp services are advertised.
3. The sale, distribution and advertisement of contraceptives.	There is no law forbidding the sale of contraceptives. Distribution of contraceptives is legally regulated. There are no firm regulations governing the country as a whole local regulations differ from town to town. Mechanical contraceptives may be advertised to the general public; Oral Contraceptives may be advertised only to health professionals (Decree 354, 1959).	In practice, the shortage of supplies of contraceptives renders the legal situation irrelevant at present. There exists a ready market for what can be obtained. Condoms and spermicides are on sale through newspaper kiosks. IUDs can be purchased irregularly in fp clinics, and in so called 'dollar shops' - for convertible currency only. With the exception of prescription contraceptives, on which 30% of the price is paid, all contraceptives must be paid for in full even from fp clinics (in national currency only). Oral contraceptives are most often dispensed through pharmacies on receipt of a physician's prescription.
4. Availability/sale of family planning related literature.	No legal impediment	While such literature is scarcely available through libraries and bookshops and fp clinics, very little material is actually available because of the shortage of paper in Poland. Until the increase of pressure group action by Church related anti-fp groups (e.g. Gaudium Vitae) newspapers and magazines provided information on contraception. Since 1979, the situation has deteriorated.

Issue	De Jure	De Facto
5. Sterilisation	Sterilisation is not legally regulated. However, 'mutilation of genital organs' is forbidden by law, and this could be theoretically applied to prevent sterilisation. An attempt to present a legal basis to Government defining sterilisation as a permissible family planning method failed due to opposition from the Church and others.	There is no demand for sterilisation as a family planning method. Nevertheless, it has been performed on those few wishing it, depending upon the willingness of the hospitals/physician concerned. However, this is done discreetly without publicity.
6. Abortion	Induced abortion is permissible within the current Abortion Act 1957 (with additional regulations from 1979 and 1981) on medical grounds irrespective of the period of pregnancy, and up to 12 weeks on socio-economic grounds. Parental consent is necessary for an abortion to be performed on a minor (under 18 years). The regulation of the Minister of Health, of January 1981 contains the following restrictions on the implementation of the Abortion Act 1957: – physicians should strive for a limitation in the number of abortions; – only specialised obstetricians and gynaecologists are allowed to issue permission for abortion, with the exception of rural areas where GPs can fulfill this role; – on request of the physician, the client must supply supporting documents to confirm grounds (e.g. statement of financial situation); – the physician should attempt to change the mind of the client, who, if persisting in the request, must sign a declaration that the medical risks are understood; – should the physician refuse to permit an abortion, the client has the right to higher appeal; – to perform an abortion in State clinics, the physician must have a 1st and 2nd degree in gynaecology. When performed in a public hospital the termination is done free of charge. It may also be paid for through privately practising physicans and their cooperatives.	Due to the shortage of contraceptives and the absence of obligatory, organised contraceptive and sex education, the number of illegal abortions is believed to have increased, in spite of the fact that the number of registered abortions has remained stable. Public opinion is generally against abortion which is regarded as a necessary evil. Up to 50% of conceptions are terminated. Up to now most restrictions remained on paper only. A large proportion of abortions have been performed in private practice and in physicians' cooperatives – where there is little legal control. In practice, physicians are so burdened with abortions that they have no time for the 'counselling' recommended in law. For example, the documentation demanded of the client's social situation may apply to State hospitals but rarely to private practitioners and cooperatives.

- 105 -

Issue	De Jure	De Facto
	Advertisement is not expressly forbidden by law.	Any attempt to advertise abortion services would be censored for political reasons to avoid offending the Church and to avoid giving the impression of the Government as officially supporting abortion.
7. Infertility treatment	There is no law covering artificial insemination.	Fertility treatment can be obtained and there is small demand; the services are supplied discreetly.
8. Sex Education/Family life education	Sex education/family life education is included in school curricula by government provision. The content is generally specified by a centrally-elaborated curriculum.	Sex education is generally implemented in elementary and secondary school. In practice the quality and quantity of sex education depends upon individual schools. Indeed, some teachers enlarge the content prescribed in the curriculum. However, the legal guidelines concerning the content of sex education courses are more often ignored, teachers often omitting sex education topics.
	Since September 1981, the subject 'Preparation for Family Life' was relegated to optional status, and, in effect, removed from the regular lesson schedule, to be taught during 'hours at the disposal of the classmaster'.	This, in effect, is a step backward, removing the obligation to provide worthwhile family life education. Sex education/family life education materials are also produced for and disseminated through: youth clubs and the mass media. Leaflets, booklets and books are published by the Polish FPA for women's groups, youth groups etc.
9. Adoption	Adoption of children is legally regulated. Only married couples may adopt. In principle, adoption is permitted to residents of Poland only. (A new law covering adoption is currently in preparation.)	No data.

Issue	De Jure	De Facto
1. Government recognition of human right to number and spacing of children (planned parenthood) Protection of family and child	The right of an individual to free choice in the number and spacing of children is specified in the Constitution 1976, Article no. 67: 'To implement by the required means the diffusion of family planning methods, and to establish the technical and legal structures to permit the exercise of planned parenthood'. Protection of family and child is also noted in the Constitution.	
2. Government and other family planning (fp) facilities/services	A Bill regulating fp facilities and services approved in March 1984, whereby the state is to provide fp services and information, is currently under consideration by the National Assembly.	Family planning services exist as part of hospital and Mother & Child Health care centres. No private fp facilities are in operation. Contraceptives at the centres are free of charge.
3. The sale, distribution and advertisement of contraceptives	The sale, distribution and advertisement of contraceptives is legally permitted.	Contraceptives may be bought at pharmacies. Orals and spermicides may be reimbursed by the National Insurance system. The IUD, condom, and diaphragm must be purchased.
4. Availability/sale of fp related literature	The sale of fp related literature is not legally forbidden.	Consumer literature is readily available from the FPA and Comissão da Condição Feminina.
5. Sterilisation	In March 1984, a Bill was passed permitting sterilisation as a method of family planning for those over 25 years. It also makes provision for non-voluntary sterilisation for mental defectives under certain circumstances. The regulations necessary to enact the law have yet to be formulated.	The regulations necessary to make the law viable have yet to be formulated. In the majority of hospitals there will be resistance from physicians to performing this surgery.
6. Abortion	In April 1984, a law permitting abortion up to 12 weeks for grave eugenic and medical reasons, and also 'ethical' reasons was approved.	The regulations necessary to make the law workable in practice have yet to be finalised. There is likely to be strong resistance to performance of abortion in public hospitals by physicians, midwives and administrators.

Issue	De Jure	De Facto
6. Abortion (contd.)		It is estimated that there may be 200,000 illegal abortions per annum based on the number of live births.
7. Infertility treatment	A law concerning artificial insemination is to be presented to Parliament.	In central hospitals good infertility services exist.
8. Sex education/family life education	A law concerning the introduction of sex education into the school curriculum was approved in March 1984.	Without the implementation of law there exists no sex education component in the curriculum. However, the Portuguese PPA provides such courses in some towns and lectures in schools by invitation from the head teacher.
9. Adoption		

Issue	De Jure	De Facto
1. Government recognition of human right to number and spacing of children (planned parenthood)	The right to determine number and spacing of children was partly introduced by decisions of the Parliament in 1938. An old law which prohibited public information of contraceptives was then annulled. At the same parliamentary session abortion was legalized in some specified cases. When the right of the women to decide herself upon abortion was introduced in 1975, it was strongly underlined that abortion must not be regarded as a family planning method but as a regrettable emergency measure when contraception has failed or has been neglected. In accordance with this view the Parliament granted significant provision for reinforcement of the public contraception services. The positive motivation for this is the ideal that every child should be a wanted child.	The use of contraceptives and the access to abortion do not, in practice, meet any obstacles from doctors, nurses and social service personnel. There are, however, still some practical and resource problems (see point 2 and 3 below). During the last ten years a new type of obstacle to the free determination of the number of children has been observed: many families do not have as many children as they really want because in most families today both parents work, by personal preference and/or by economic necessity. That is regarded as one of the reasons for the low birthrate. Every woman bears on average 1.6 children. She would have to bear 2.1 children in order to reproduce her generation. The low birthrate has earlier been regarded as positive with regard to the population of the world. Today it is regarded both by the public opinion and by the politicians as, in the long run, a threat to the survival of Swedish society.
Protection of family and child	This is guaranteed by the Social Services Act 1981. Sexual intercourse with a minor under 15 years is an offence, if the partners are not of about the same age and degree of maturity.	
2. Government and other family planning (fp) facilities/services	Family planning is regulated by the law according to the directives and subsidies described above. Advertising of fp services is not legally regulated.	Government subsidies are used to encourage expansion of contraceptive advisory services. The public health or other organisation providing these services receive a grant through the public health insurance system. The requirement for the grant is that the consultation must be free of charge to the person seeking advice and that contraceptives, to some extent, be dispensed free of charge. Diaphragms or IUDs inserted during the consultation are free. Condoms and chemical preparations in limited quantities may also be dispensed on such consultations. Oral contraceptives are sold under the same discount system as other medicines.

- 109 -

Issue	De Jure	De Facto
		A system of family planning services integrated with the maternity health care system has been built up. Free counselling is available at maternity clinics, through private physicians and through the Swedish PPA.
		At about 30 locations there are special centres where young people can obtain advice on different methods of fp. Midwives are also trained to give advice on contraception. Midwives can also give gynaecological examinations, insert IUDs and prescribe oral contraceptives.
		The number of visits to the contraceptive advisory services per 1,000 women aged 15-44 increased 1975-1981 by 41%, from 249 to 351 visits annually. The real need is estimated to 500 visits.
		A public commission in 1983 published a report (with an English summary) on the implementation of the abortion law of 1975. The commission found that the extended and improved contraceptive advisory services have strongly contributed to stabilising the number of abortions since the introduction of free abortion in 1975. The commission does not believe that the incidence of abortion has been reduced, mostly because of the fact that so many pregnancies occur in spite of a rational use of contraception. At the same time the commission points to a number of further possible improvements of contraceptive advice, of public information and of sex education in the schools.
3. The Sale, advertisement	distribution and of contraceptives	No legal regulation forbids the sale and advertisement of contraceptives. The distribution of contraceptives is legally regulated. An Ordinance of 1970 provides that contraceptives must be sold under hygienic conditions. Oral contraceptives are under the Pharmaceutical Products Decree and may only be distributed through pharmacies. IUDs are normally distributed by the manufacturer to the physician. Oral contraceptives require the prescription of a physician or a midwife.
		See also under 2. All contraceptives are distributed through contraceptive advisory services, hospitals and private doctors - condoms only in small quantities. These are mostly distributed on the open market. The reason for this is the judgement that this is the most effective form of distribution for this special type of contraceptive. Thus condoms are easily available today. They are sold in petrol stations, department stores, supermarkets, kiosks and newspaper stands among others.

- 110 -

Issue	De Jure	De Facto
4. Availability/sale of family planning (fp) related literature	There is no law restricting the availability/sale of fp related literature.	Consumer literature is readily available, and can be obtained from family planning clinics, bookshops, libraries and RFSU.
5. Sterilisation	Sterilisation is legally regulated. In January 1976 a Sterilisation Act came into effect, as a complement to other laws on birth control. The Act states that sterilisation is available to both men and women over the age of 25 (if Swedish citizens) as a method of family planning. The operation must be preceded by counselling.	Up to 1981 2.3% of Swedish women and men aged 20-44 had been sterilized.
	No public agency may take the initiative for a sterilisation.	Dissatisfaction and regret after the operation has been observed in a few cases. As sterilisation is conducted in public hospitals advertising is irrelevant.
6. Abortion	Abortion is legally regulated (1975 Act; see above), and available on request up to the 18th week of pregnancy. No grounds are specified which would limit access to abortion. If a woman requests an abortion she is entitled to have this performed, having first consulted a doctor up to the 12th week of pregnancy. After the 12th week up to the 18th week, the abortion is allowed after the woman has also consulted a welfare officer.	The Abortion Act of 1975 is fully implemented without obstacles. As abortion is freely available and conducted free of charge in public hospitals there are no illegal abortions. Advertising does not exist.
	After the 18th week, an abortion is allowed only if there are especially compelling reasons and approval has been obtained from the National Board of Health and Welfare. Approval shall not be granted if the foetus is viable. The women must be a Swedish citizen or domiciled in Sweden. A women contemplating an abortion must always be offered the counselling services of a welfare officer; this counselling is optional and should be	
	aimed, not at influencing the women's decision, but at helping her to arrive at a decision with which she herself will be satisfied.	
	The same conditions apply to minors.	

Issue	De Jure	De Facto
7. Infertility treatment	Artificial insemination is permitted but not legally regulated in detail. An expert appointed by the government in 1983 proposed that a husband who has agreed to artificial insemination by a donor of his wife will be the legal father of the offspring, with all subsequent obligations.	It is predicted that because anonymity cannot be guaranteed, donors will be less likely to come forward, seeking treatment elsewhere.
	From 1985, all children have the right to know the identity of their biological father.	Until 1985, infertility treatment services has been widely available from women's clinics, hospitals, and through obstetric and gynaecological services in private practice throughout Sweden. However, the new law may lead to the closure of private establishments offeringthe service.
	Artificial insemination may only be performed in a public hospital.	Both diagnosis and treatment are accepted within the public health insurance system which means low costs for those seeking advice.
	The idea of an elite bank for insemination is rejected by the experts.	
	Legislation concerning in vitro fertilization is being prepared. It will probably prohibit the transplanting of a fertilized egg for another woman's uterus with the intention of delivering the baby to the woman who produced the egg. On the other hand it will certainly be allowed to replant a fertilized egg in the uterus of the woman who produced the egg.	
8. Sex education/family life education	Sex education/family life education has been included in the school curriculum by Government provision since 1942. The first goal of sex education is formulated as follows in the guidelines adopted by the Government: 'The pupils are to acquire a knowledge of anatomy, physiology, psychology, ethics and social relations calculated to improve their prospects of achieving interpersonal relations characterised by responsibility, consideration and care for their fellow beings, and in this way experiencing sexuality as a source of happiness together with another person'.	Sex education is implemented at all levels of education, though least developed at the nursery school level. A handbook for dealing with sex problems and answering quetions at this level was published by the Swedish PPA in 1983. A handbook for sex education in the whole school system was published by the Central Board of Education in 1977 as a result of a ten year public commission work. A full English translation of the handbook (300 pages) is available. The individual school/teacher has great freedom in deciding the content of the sex education provided, within the frames of the handbook. Investigations have indicated that practically all pupils get sex education; however, the quantity and quality varies. Basic training for teachers in sex education is (contd).

Issue	De Jure	De Facto
		practically nonexistent, although in-service training is sometimes good.
9. Adoption	Adoption is legally permissible to those over 24 years old. (In special cases to younger people.) Both couples and individuals may adopt, always after testing of their ability by the social welfare committee and in the law courts. The adopted child has the right to full social benefits.	Up to the middle of this century mostly children of single and distressed Swedish mothers were adopted by childless couples; in the forties and fifties 1,000 children annually. After this time these cases have become less and less usual because of better contraceptive technique, legalisation of abortion and improved public assistance. Today the great majority of the adoptees are foreign.
		In 1982 about 1,500 foreign children were adopted, often by families who already had children of their own. The number was considerably higher some years ago. Today there is a slight decrease. If the children are adopted at an early age their integration in Swedish society seems to be unproblematic.

Issue	De Jure	De Facto
1. Government recognition of human right to number and spacing of children (planned parenthood)	The right of the individual to free determination of the number and spacing of children is guaranteed by the 1983 Constitution which updates the Family Planning Act 1965: 'Individuals may have as many children as they want and when they want'. This represents a sanction for the use of contraceptives.	Since promulgation of the law, different governments took different stands on the subject, which hindered the effective provision of family planning services. The present government has taken a staunch antinatalist stand but education and distribution of contraceptives and of clinical services are still not at the desired level.
Protection of family and child	This is also guaranteed by the Constitution and a special family law.	This cannot be done very effectively under existing social and economic conditions.
2. Government and other family planning (fp) facilities/services	Family planning is legally regulated and corresponding services are set up within the public health services. It is legally permitted to advertise these services. A law of 1983 empowers nurses and midwives to provide contraceptive services.	Family planning services exist as part of State hospitals and Mother & Child Health care (MCH) centres. Contraceptives are free of charge. The centres also cater for private fee-paying family planning consultation. When provided in state hospitals and MCH centres, these services are free but only about 50% are able to provide it due to lack of personnel and equipment. Service distribution throughout Turkey remains uneven.
3. The sale, distribution, and advertisement of contraceptives	There is no law prohibiting the sale of contraceptives, though their distribution is governed by law.	Distribution has not been systematised and remains unsatisfactory.
4. Availability/sale of fp related literature	There is no law forbidding the sale of fp related literature.	FP related literature is available from fp centres, bookshops, libraries, and the Turkish FPA itself.
5. Sterilisation	A law of April 1983 specifies the legal conditions allowing voluntary sterilisation, making it available on request to those aged 18 or over, if there are no medical contraindications. For those who are married, the consent of the spouse is necessary.	Clinics are still in the establishment stage and de facto information not available.
6. Abortion	The Law of 1983 allows abortion on request during the first 10 weeks of pregnancy. After 10 weeks, termination of pregnancy is permitted under two conditions: if it threatens or might threaten the life of the mother; or if the child or its offspring might be seriously handicapped. A report by two specialists (one in Obstetrics & Gynecology, the other in a related field) would be required to certify the	Same as for item 5.

- 114 -

Issue	De Jure	De Facto
	existence of these conditions.	
	In cases of emergency, when an immediate termination is necessary, a qualified doctor can perform an abortion.	
	The husband's consent is a necessary condition for the termination of pregnancy of married women. For minors, the consent of a parent or guardian and that of a magistrate's court is necessary.	
7. Infertility treatment	No legal regulation exists to cover this treatment.	Generally provided in hospitals as a standard treatment.
8. Sex education/family life education	No legal regulation covers the provision of sex education in schools.	Sex education is not included in the school curriculum at any level. It is treated to some degree in the mass media.
		Radio news broadcast announced in September that "Population Planning" courses will be given in secondary education as of this school year.
9. Adoption	The adoption of children is dealt with by a separate law which specifies that adopters must be over 40 years of age and at least 18 years older than the adoptee. A child may be adopted only by a couple who have no children than their own.	No data.

Issue	De Jure	De Facto
1. Government recognition of human right to number and spacing of children (planned parenthood)	Not legally or otherwise specified. (The UK has no written constitution).	In practice, the existing laws (eg. the NHS act 1973) may be seen to constitute Government's recognition of/commitment to the human right to planned parenthood, free choice in individual determination of the number and spacing of children, and the protection of the family and child. This position is reflected, in practice.
Protection of family and child	Indirect: through other laws.	
2. Government and other family planning (fp) facilities/services	FP facilities and services are legally regulated through the National Health Service (NHS) Reorganisation Act, 1973. This law extended the provisions of the previous NHS family planning acts by empowering and obliging local health authorities to make arrangements for giving advice, medical examinations, contraceptive services and treatments (including sterilisation), and contraceptive supplies to those seeking them. It also makes FP services free under the NHS.	Both public and private FP facilities exist. Government (NHS) services are offered through hospitals, MCH institutions, domiciliary services, general practitioners and FP clinics. Some separate services exist for adolescents. While the general availability of the NHS services means that very few women would resort to private fp consultation, clinics, which offer the best range of fp services, and which are cheaper to run, are suffering from lack of adequate funding in the economic recession. Insufficient opening times in some areas are forcing women to GPs, who often dispense only orals.
	The law allows for the advertisement of FP clinics but restrictions are imposed in accordance with the codes of advertising authorites.	The original NHS Family Planning Act (1967) received support from commercial TV which decided that it would be reasonable in future to accept advertising of official and officially sponsored FP advisory services, from central Government, local authorities, the FPA, and other voluntary bodies cooperating with local authorities in providing such advisory services in local clinics.
3. The sale, distribution and advertisement of contraceptives	There is no legal prohibition of the sale of contraceptives, though their sale/distribution is legally regulated.	Contraceptives and services (eg. sterilisation) are free of charge under the NHS, with the exception of condoms which are available from NHS clinics alone.
	There are no legal limitations on the sale of condoms, though local by-laws in some areas may prohibit their sale from vending machines in public places.	Contraceptives and services may also be purchased within the private sector. Cost is not believed to be an obstacle to use, except to some young people.

Issue	De Jure	De Facto
	Sale and distribution (issue) of oral contraceptives, on prescription only, through pharmacies, FP clinics, and some medical practitioners.	In practice, IUDs are supplied/inserted by medical practitioners and properly trained nurses in clinics/surgeries.
	IUDs are not covered by the Medicines Act as they are considered 'appliances'. They may soon be subject to licensing as a medicinal product.	Contraceptives are advertised in some newspapers and magazines. Their acceptance on TV, radio and some public places, however, is limited. In practice, anti-family planning pressure group and professional resistance ensures that effective contraceptive advertising is limited.
	The law allows for the advertisement of contraceptives; there are no specific injunctions so long as the advertisements do not contravene the provisions of the Indecent Advertisements Act (1959) and the Unsolicited Goods and Services Act (1971) which makes it a criminal offence to send unsolicited matter through the post describing sexual technique. Some controls on the advertisement of contraceptives can be made under the terms of the Medicines Act (Sect. 45/1) which gives the Govt. the power to prohibit advertisements relating to specific medical products or which are likely to lead to the use of such products.	The Independent Broadcasting Authority bans brand-name advertising of contraceptives.
	Additionally, further restrictions/limitations/controls may be imposed by the Advertising Standards Authority and the Independent Broadcasting Authority's Code of Advertising Standards and Practice.	Pregnancy test advertisements are controlled in this manner - the advertisement may state only the service provided, the fee, request for a sample, and for the person to state their age. The ASA checks advertisements with its medical advisers and local services. The Independent Broadcasting Authority (IBA) has banned advertisements for pregnancy testing services.
	The Pharmaceutical Society's Statement upon Matters of Professional Conduct contains no reference to contraceptives. Para. 5., however, states that 'the appearance of the premises should reflect the professional character of the pharmacy' which would not, it is said, preclude 'a discreet display of contraceptives'.	

Issue	De Jure	De Facto
4. Availability/sale of family planning (fp) related literature	There is nothing in the law which forbids the sale or dissemination of FP-related literature.	Consumer literature is available and can be obtained from FP clinics, in many hospitals, from family physicians (GPs), in some libraries and Citizens' Advice Bureaux. In the near future it will also be available through consenting pharmacies. The actual availability of consumer literature varies in different parts of the country.
5. Sterilisation	Legal regulations on sterilisation were specifically included in Sect. 4 of the NHS Reorganisation Act (1973) Female sterilisation was excluded from the 1967 Act. Sterilisation is legal on grounds of health or transmission of disease, and as a family planning method for both males and females.	In some regions of the UK, NHS sterilisation facilities are lacking or insufficient to meet the demand. Sterilisation is available however to those willing to travel to another area and/or to pay for the service in the private sector. Under the NHS, the service is free of charge.
6. Abortion	Abortion is legally regulated under the 1967 Abortion Act, and is permissible on medical and socio-medical grounds. Under the Act, an abortion is permitted where two medical practitioners believe in good faith, that continuation of pregnancy would involve greater risk to the physical or mental health of the mother or her children than if the pregnancy were terminated. Account may be taken of the mother's actual or foreseeable environment. An abortion may also be performed if the practitioners believe that there is substantial risk that the child may be seriously handicapped by physical or mental abnormalities.

Abortion is permitted up to 28 weeks, free of charge under NHS. The law applies to minors, but girls under 16 years required written consent of parents, guardian, or social worker if they are in care. | About 50% of abortions performed in Britain are carried out under the NHS, the remainder being done privately. Legal abortions are performed in both hospitals and outpatient clinics.

In 1983 the cost of an abortion in a private clinic (situated in major cities) was around £120.

While some will find few obstacles in such centres, it is known that the free public services are sometimes dominated by unsympathetic physicians who may obstruct access to abortion. |

Issue	De Jure	De Facto
	Advertisement of abortion is not expressly forbidden by law.	Restrictions on the advertisement of abortion had been imposed by the advertising authorities in their codes of standards and practice. In practice, abortion advertisements are rare in the media, though there are public displays (posters) advertising abortion services (eg Pregnancy Advisory Service).
7. Infertility Treatment	At present there are no legal regulations covering AID/infertility, although the Royal College of Obstetricians and Gynaecologists have issued guidelines governing the practice, and pre-requisites for AID (October 1976). There is at present much discussion of the legal issues involved in AID (e.g. legitimacy of children, paternity etc.). At present it is permitted, including in the case of a married couple if neither furnishes grounds for divorce on the basis of unreasonable conduct (provided it is carried out with the husbands' permission), and if it is not construed as adultery by either recipient or donor.	Infertility treatment is selectively available within the NHS from hospitals. However, in some regions there are long waiting lists.
8. Sex education/family life education	There is no government provision for the inclusion of sex education/family life education in the school curriculum, merely a recommendation that such education be provided in an appropriate form.	The actual inclusion of sex education/ family life education in school curricula varies widely, though the majority of secondary schools in the UK do offer some direction to pupils. The quality of what is imparted varies widely, and is not generally comprehensive. The content is decided by the head of the school in which it is offered. This teaching is given in some youth clubs and rarely through the mass media. Publications on the subject are widely available for all age-groups.
9. Adoption	No legal steps can be taken, before a baby is 6 weeks old, to permit the mother to make any decision about adoption. In 1982, a delayed provision of the 1982 Childrens' Act came into force and it became illegal for adoptions to be to be made by private individuals. The agreement to adopt must be signed by the mother in the presence of a magistrate and also by the father if she is married. Once the order is made the child stands in exactly the same relationship to his/her adoptive parents as a natural child (reinheritance).	There are many more people now longing to adopt than there are babies 'available for adoption'. Unwanted, (white) healthy babies theoretically no longer exist. Adoption figures show a spectacular fall in the last 12 years, from a peak of 24,831 in 1968 to 10,609 in 1980.

Issue	De Jure	De Facto
1. Government recognition of human right to number and spacing of children (planned parenthood)	The Yugoslav Constitution of 1974 established the human right to decide freely on the number and spacing of children and decreed that this right may be restricted only for health reasons (Art. 191). Identical provisions are embodied in the Constitutions of all Federal Units (i.e., the six Republics and two autonomous provinces). After 1974, elaboration and legal regulation of this principle became the exclusive jurisdiction of the Federal Units.	Statutory elaboration of the Constitutional principle by the Federal Units has only been partially completed to date. A number of the Federal Units have not yet enacted all relevant and required legislation to ensure full implementation of the Constitutional guarantees. Slovenia and Croatia are the two most advanced Republics in this regard.
Protection of family and child	Protection of the family and child is also guaranteed in the Constitutions at Federal and Republic/Provincial levels. This principle is supported directly by special family law and indirectly through other laws enacted by the Federal Units in accordance with their exclusive jurisdiction over family relationships. While these laws must respect the Constitutional principle noted above, they may be adjusted according to prevailing local conditions. Separate laws and regulations variously exist to deal with the health and welfare of children (e.g., education, upbringing, health and social protection, child allowances, etc) and the health and other protection of the mother.	The social community offers protection, services and assistance to married and unmarried couples, natural and adopted children. Legal regulation of family relationships, in which decisions on childbirth are deemed a crucial aspect, is still underway in the Federal Units and not yet far advanced. In only two Republics (Slovenia and Croatia) have integral and all-embracing family codes been enacted, statutorily regulating marriage, parent-child relationships, adoptions, etc.

Issue	De Jure	De Facto
2. Government and other family planning (fp) facilities/services	Family planning facilities and services, including those for abortion, are legally regulated by the Federal Units in accordance with Art, 191 of the Constitution. Since 1968 contraception has been an integral part of compulsory (minimal) public health protection services regulated by Republic and Provincial legislation on health insurance.	Government, but not private, fp facilities exist as part of hospitals, Mother & Child Health care clinics and other public health institutions where medical services are provided.
	The advertisement of FP clinics is not permitted by law, though since 1960, pregnant women seeking abortion are required by law to be informed of the contraceptive services by all public health institutions.	
Protection of family and child	Since 1974, laws adopted by the Federal Units devote several provisions to assuring men and women of all appropriate measures and forms of health protection related to contraception, and most specify the types and minimal requirements of health and institutions, organisations and facilities authorised and empowered to provide FP/contraceptive services.	The community offers protection, services and assistance to married and unmarried couples.
3. The sale, distribution and advertisement of contraceptives.	The law does not allow for the advertisement of medical contraceptives.	
	Their manufacture, import and sale are not forbidden unless so specified in the Drug Marketing Act.	Yugoslavia manufactures contraceptives but local condoms are said to be of poor quality. Foreign currency problems have restricted imports.
	There is no law governing the distribution of contraceptives, but oral contraceptives and IUDs are available only on medical prescription from an authorised gynaecologist and consultation with a health worker, is obligatory. Barrier contraceptives are available without prescription or medical consultation.	Condoms are not available from vending machines. Due to the restrictions on contraceptive imports, some types of contraceptives, previously imported, are reported to be in short supply (e.g. diaphragms).
		Oral contraceptives and IUDs are free of charge on prescription. Condoms are available and sold in street booths, tobacco shops, pharmacies, etc.

- 121 -

Issue	De Jure	De Facto
4. Availability/sale of family planning (fp) related literature	By law, relevant institutions are directed to produce sex education literature	Numerous books, manuals, leaflets are available, eg. in fp counselling centres.
5. Sterilisation	Legal regulations on sterilisation are in force in only two Federal Units - Croatia and Slovenia. Both are similar in permitting sterilisation for medical reasons at any age, and as an fp method for males and females over 35 years of age. In both Republics sterilisation may be carried out only at the request of the person to be sterilised and written consent must be included with the request. For minors, the right of a parent or guardian to request sterilisation on behalf of the person they represent is regulated in detail. All general, clinical and specialised hospitals with organised gynecological, obstetric or surgical services (and in Croatia, for men, hospitals with urological ward) are authorised to perform sterilisations. All other health organisations must obtain special authorisation from the Republic's designated health authority. In Croatia, health organisations must report all sterilisations carried out to the health records agency within 30 days. The Croatian law also stipulates that when sterilisation is carried out as an independent medical operation, the costs are borne by the applicant insofar as the self-management interest community for health has not statutorily decreed otherwise.	The legal situation is reportedly reflected in practice, but the number of sterilisations carried out is negligible.
6. Abortion	The legal regulation of abortion in all republics is enacted on the basis of the Constitutional position on the free determination of the number and spacing of children. Induced abortion up to the 10th week is permitted, on request, providing there is no risk to health. Abortion after the 10th week is permitted with the consent of a medical commission. Reasons for permission include: medical, ethical, and personal, family and financial reasons. If at first the request for termination after the 10th week is refused by the commission, an appeal procedure may be employed.	Medical services implement fully the legal statutes, though illegal abortion is not unknown, due to the medical complications which come to light through hospitals. However, they are thought to be small in number considering the relatively liberal law.

Issue	De Jure	De Facto
	Special conditions govern a request for abortion from minors (namely consent of parents who have been informed of health consequences).	Abortion continues to play a major role in fertility regulation in Yugoslavia, with the numbers equalling or even surpassing the number of live births, depending on the province. A decline in the number of abortions since 1967 is believed to be the result of improvements in the work of the health service covering contraceptive services. More clinics are in operation and a wider variety of contraceptives have been made available.
7. Infertility treatment	No data.	No data.
8. Sex education/family life education	This subject is legally included within the school curriculum for all levels of schooling, and across a range of subjects.	Implementation of sex education in school, in practice, depends upon the willingness and integrity of teachers. Sex education is also taught in special courses in youth clubs and colleges. It is also addressed by the mass media.
9. Adoption	Adoption is legally regulated (1971/74). Republic and provincial laws cover conditions for adoption, relations between adopter and adoptee, right to inherit etc.	No data.

Key:

Austria	A
Belgium	B
Denmark	DK
Federal Republic of Germany	D
Finland	SF
France	F
German Democratic Republic	DDR
Hungary	H
Ireland	IRL
Italy	I
Netherlands	NL
Norway	N
Poland	PL
Portugal	P
Sweden	S
Turkey	TR
United Kingdom	UK
Yugoslavia	YU

With the aim of 'surveying the current situation relating to the fulfilment of human rights', the preceding tabular presentation of de jure and de facto data covering 9 planned parenthood issues presents a relatively objective picture of 18 national situations. Although the data must speak for itself as an indication of government commitment to planned parenthood rights, it is nevertheless possible to crudely evaluate the state of planned parenthood provision in most of Europe.

The nominal commitment of governments to the international resolutions, reviewed on page 47 of this report, implies that states are obliged to:

1. Legally or constitutionally recognise the right of an individual to decide freely and responsibly on the number and spacing of her/his children;

2. Enable the individual to exercise her/his right by providing or facilitating access to: information,

education, and services (including contraceptives).

The summary evaluation following is based on a country by country assessment of whether: firstly, legislation is currently in existence which has the overall effect of enabling/facilitating the free exercise of planned parenthood (as defined by the working group)(1); and secondly, government involvement in the provision of specific services/facilities is sufficient to be regarded as fulfilling condition 2 above.

ISSUE 1: **Government recognition of the human right to determine the number and spacing of children (within the context of its responsibilities for the protection of family and child).**

Portugal, Turkey and Yugoslavia are exceptional insofar as the human right to family planning is explicitly recorded in their Constitutions. Of the 18 countries in the survey, Constitutional recognition of this right is implied in a further 6 (A, F, I, NL, N, S). Moreover, national legal anomalies aside (for example the lack of a constitution in the UK), government recognition, de jure, is in evidence in 6 other countries (DK, D, DDR, H, Pl, UK). That is to say that in these countries there exists legislation which effectively guarantees the populations the right of access to planned parenthood, even though this may not be formally stated in human rights terms, or necessarily reflected in the situation, de facto.

Extending the analysis to the de facto situations, it may be noted that in a total of 12 countries (A, DK, F, D, DDR, H, NL, N, PL, S, TR, UK, YU), the state is so involved in the provision of planned parenthood services that it may be assumed that there is reasonable government recognition

---

(1) It is recognised that certain 'restrictive' legislation can have a valid purpose to protect individuals against health risks, etc., rather than curtail their rights, and therefore still qualify as having the sum effect of facilitating the (responsible) exercise of planned parenthood. Of course, this is not to say that restrictive legislation designated by governments as protecting the best interests of the individual, parent, or society can be accepted as such.

of this human right at least as far as overall contraceptive services provision is concerned (though abortion services produce anomalies).

However, this number excludes certain states which may have de jure recognition but which are believed to display inadequate government support for services such that a minimum exercise of such rights is a practical possibility for the majority of citizens in need (eg. Portugal, Italy).

In 16 countries there is evidence of significant government support for all or the majority of planned parenthood issues, whether they are recognised, de jure, or not. This excludes Ireland, where little state recognition has been forthcoming either de jure or de facto.

ISSUE 2: **Family planning facilities/services**

The significance of the legal regulation of family planning facilities is threefold:

- prohibitive/repressive;
- protective (regulations covering the dispensing/ administration of medical preparations);
- enabling/ensuring that family planning provision is sufficient to satisfy demand.

In Ireland, alone, the legal regulation of family planning facilities is prohibitive/repressive, aiming to deter (with limited success) the non-married sector of the population.

Protective legislation covering family planning facilities, exists in one form or another, in all of the participating countries.

Legal regulation to ensure nationwide provision exists in 11 countries (DK, SF, F, D, I, PL, P, S, TR, UK, YU). However, in France, Italy, Portugal and Turkey the assistance of the state is not uniform for all regions. In addition, in Austria, DDR, Netherlands, Norway and Hungary, the governments make the effort to guarantee demand, in practice, without resort to legislation.

ISSUE 3: **The sale, distribution and advertisement of contraceptives**

Legislation relating to this issue overlaps with issue 2 on the subject of distribution. The question here concerns whether the state facilitates or impedes, through law and/or practice, public access to methods. Concerning the sale of contraceptives, legislation is on the whole protective rather than repressive. Laws covering advertising can also be interpreted as protective (of public sensitivities, morality, physical safety, and against unjustifiable commercial profit).

In this area, the absence of law is on the whole to be interpreted positively in human rights terms.

With the exception of Ireland, there are no legal impediments as such in the remaining 17 countries, outside of protective regulatory provisions to cover the medical risks of oral contraceptive provision, and the insertion of IUDs.

Concerning the advertising of contraceptives, with the exception of Ireland (where there is total legal prohibition) and France (where the advertising of brand names is prohibited), no legal regulation exists in the remaining countries(2) on general advertising, with the exception of prescription methods (orals and IUDs). Regulations covering appropriate media for such methods, and the conditions of their advertising are protective of public safety rather than restrictive/repressive(3).

The relevance of the de facto situation relating to this issue vis-à-vis the legal situation is whether governments impose, or permit the imposition of, any non-legal impediments to the free sale, advertising and distribution of contraceptives, or actively facilitate it.

Where availability of contraceptives more or less meets demand, the situation in many countries is that there is neither special help from governments (for example with the purchase of contraceptives), nor any impediment: for example in Austria, Denmark, Netherlands, Norway, and Sweden. Partial assistance is provided in Finland, where the first three months of oral contraceptives are free of charge. Much more extensive assistance is provided in the UK, Yugoslavia, Hungary, and the DDR, where most or all contraceptives are either 'free' (i.e. available within the national health systems) or heavily subsidised. Significant governmental/legal impediments to the

---

(2) No data on Turkey
(3) Note: Restrictions on advertising of contraceptives may still be imposed by non-governmental sources, e.g. media authorities.

distribution of contraceptives remain in Ireland, though they have recently been relaxed in the case of condoms and spermicides.

An economic impediment to contraceptive production and importation exists in Poland which impedes accessibility due to the national economic crisis; and in France family planning clinics are restricted to the issue of prescriptions rather than supplies (except in the case of minors requesting anonymity), though the cost of oral contraceptives and IUDs is reimbursed by social security.

In spite of the <u>de jure</u> situation, in France, Italy, Turkey, Portugal, Poland and the FRG there is inadequate governmental assistance to contraceptors (for different reasons) considering the need for it.

ISSUE 4: **Availability of family planning related literature**

This is not an area in which governmental regulations or conditions are likely to be imposed where commercial production of literature appears to satisfy demand. The PPA is often empowered and financially assisted by governments to fill any gaps in provision. It is not possible here to discern if this is sufficient.

No government, <u>with the exception of Ireland</u>, imposes any legal impediment on the availability of family planning related literature (though some governments (e.g. in D, UK) have been known to attempt to influence the content of PPA-produced literature. Certain governments (Austria, Belgium) leave the supply of such literature to the commercial sector.

The availability of literature from whatever source is likely to reflect the availability or non-availability of services.

ISSUE 5: **Sterilisation**

The legal status of this issue, as distinct from general and professional medical attitudes to it as a method of family planning, will determine whether access to it should be regarded as a basic human right in any single country. Where legal regulations are permissive and enabling they are likely to contain protective regulations covering age of consent and the place in which the operation can be (safely) conducted. The legally designated age of consent/responsibility differs widely and it is an open question whether such age limits could be regarded simply as 'protective' law or as infringements of human rights.

In the absence of specific laws covering sterilisation, there are legal statutes which could be brought to bear in FRG, France, Belgium, Hungary, Italy and Poland, to challenge the legality of this operation as a method of fertility regulation. These usually concern the non-legality of mutilation of the body for purposes unrelated to illness.

Sterilisation is a legally recognised method of family planning in 10 countries (with minimum age limits where legally specified): A, DK (25+), SF (18+), DDR (women only), N (25+), P (25+), S (25+), TR (18+), UK, YU (35+, Croatia and Slovenia only). However, of the above there is medical professional resistance noted in Austria, DDR and Yugoslavia; and financial impediments such as exclusion from health insurance reimbursement for family planning in Belgium, Austria, France and Italy. Medical and other health professional resistance to the implementation of law is noted in a total of 10 countries in all.

The government actively facilitates access to sterilisation as a method of family planning in 8 countries: DK, F, NL, N, P (1984 law), S, TR and UK. In France, sterilisation is unrecognised as a method of contraception both at the legal and practical level.

ISSUE 6: **Abortion**

Where enabling legislation exists on abortion, there are regulations which specify age of consent and the necessity of counselling. If women have difficulty in fulfilling criteria for abortion, even though it is theoretically legal on request, then it cannot be said that there is sufficient government support for abortion as a right in practice.

Abortion is available on social or socio-medical grounds, with a time limit, in 15 countries: A, DK, SF, F, D, DDR, H, IRL, NL, P, PL, S, TR, UK, YU. It is totally forbidden in Ireland and Belgium. In Portugal an abortion law has recently been formulated.

Abortion is available on request, within specified time limits, without the consent of physicians in 8 countries: A, DK, DDR, F, N, S, TR, YU.

Abortion is available on request, within specified time limits, with the consent of physicians and with the fulfillment of certain conditions (e.g. socio-economic grounds) in 7 countries: SF, D, H, IRL, NL, PL, UK.

Government reimbursement for abortion (within state health systems) is available in 9 countries: DK, SF, DDR, H, N, NL, S, UK, YU.

No government assistance is available in 7 countries: A, D, I, NL, PL, TR. Assistance (through the social security system) may become available in Netherlands and Turkey through legal changes in progress.

ISSUE 7: Infertility treatment

Legislation exists concerning infertility treatment in 2 countries: Yugoslavia and Hungary. This is protective and enabling in nature, concerning the rights of children born of AID procedures. Similar kinds of legislation are under preparation in other countries, though at present, 16 countries are without formal legislation in this area. The right to such a service is legally enshrined in the majority of countries within other health service legislation.

Limited government assistance, through health services, is available in A, B, F, D, DDR, SF, H, I, NL, N, PL, S, TR, UK, YU. No data is available for Italy and Portugal. For most countries, infertility treatment is not available in all regions.

In general, it appears that enabling legislation is not necessarily required to cover this treatment as a basic human right, if it is available as part of the general health services. On the other hand there is little indication of governmental support on any large scale, considering the pronatalist concerns of so many of these governments and the rate of potential infertility/sub-fertility in any single country. It may thus be regarded as a neglected dimension in terms of government support for the human right to planned parenthood.

ISSUE 8: Sex education/family life education (FLE)

Legislation and practice on this subject displays a great reluctance by many governments to promote the human right of the population to information/education on family planning and sexuality. Where a nationally standardised curriculum has been designed there is still little realistic effort at the national/state level to see that this curriculum can be effectively implemented. There are several reasons for this. Firstly, unlike in mathematics or biology, with few exceptions there is no consensus on what should be taught in such a value-laden area. Because of this, secondly, there is little incentive at the teacher- training level to 'educate the educators'. Finally, there is an unwillingness on the part of most national governments to risk unpopularity by promoting a single value position on the pedagogy of sex education.

Consequently, the majority of governments, in one way or another, 'opt out' of direct promotion of this right. For example, not one country report recognises that there is a satisfactory standard of education in sexual and contraceptive matters in their schools at all levels. Only Sweden can declare that comprehensive assistance in this area is forthcoming from government. Partial assistance is recognised in Denmark, Hungary and Finland.

There exists legal provision for sex education/FLE (including some established definition of what it entails) in 9 countries: A, D, SF, F, DDR, H, N, S, Y., with such legislation imminent in Netherlands and Portugal. In the remainder, the subject is either totally ignored, or receives so little attention at the national level as to be irrelevant.

This situation raises the question: what powers do governments have at their disposal to improve the situations - even if they were willing - in the light of the relative autonomy which schools have on what instruction is provided?

ISSUE 9:   **Adoption**

All legislation relating to adoption is protective/ enabling in nature (of the rights of the adopter/adoptee). Impediments to the 'right' to adopt stem from causes outside of government legislation/practice: most often a shortage of children to adopt. Legislation of this kind above exists in all the countries. Thirteen countries identify lack of adoptees as the major problem in this area. There is a lack of data on the practical situation in 5 countries. Government assistance in the supervision of the adoption process is recorded in 8 countries.

COUNTRY CASE STUDIES

The objectives of the 5 country case studies are as follows:

-to furnish an historical/political background to the formulation of existing planned parenthood laws in the countries concerned, in order to better understand the positive or negative role these laws play in the provision of services and facilities;

-to identify the relative involvement of government vis-à-vis other relatively independent professional, bureaucratic or other power groups in the implementation of laws as they stand;

-to provide a PPA perspective on the relative quality of planned parenthood law and services/facilities, with recommendations to their government and non-governmental authorities to correct what are seen as shortcomings in the current situation.

Chapter Six

COUNTRY CASE STUDIES

Planned Parenthood Legislation and Practice in Belgium
F Deven

Introduction

This paper aims to document patterns, trends and developments relating to the legal and de facto situation of planned parenthood in Belgium. This refers more specifically to fertility regulation and sex/family life education. Therefore, an attempt is made to grasp the socio-economic and cultural roots which characterised Belgian society in the past and the influence they have at present.

An overview is made of the current legislation relating to fertility regulation and sex/family life education. Subsequently, the fertility and fertility-regulating behaviour of the population is documented. Use is made of census data, empirical data from the (national) surveys on family development, and of information from opinion polls.

Events and developments influencing the planned parenthood situation will be dealt with in more detail. Particular attention is paid to the abortion issue as its legal and the factual situations display the greatest variation.

Throughout the account, an attempt is made to point to some general dynamics with a view to providing recommendations for policy-making on planned parenthood issues.

Context and conditions

Within an area of 11,400 square miles, Belgium had in 1830 approximately 3.8 million inhabitants. The population grew to 7 million by the turn of the century and to nearly ten million in 1981. Although it is still divided into nine provinces, the division into regions and communities has become more significant. Accordingly, two major (linguistic) communities can be distinguished:

the Flemish (Vlaamse Gemeenschap) and the Francophone (Communauté Française). The former - Flanders - holds about 57% of the Belgian population; the latter - Wallonia - about 32%. From the socio-linguistic point of view, the area of the capital (Brussel/Bruxelles) should be distinguished, holding 10% of the population. Finally, it has to be noted that the Walloon region includes a German-speaking community, comprising 0.7% of the Belgian population.

The country may be characterised in the nineteenth and in the first half of the twentieth century by a high degree of heterogeneity: cultural, economic and social. In addition, wide variation occurred in demographic trends (fertility rates, infant mortality rates, and life expectancy at birth). These differentials within the emerging state of Belgium may be understood in part by a clearly different pattern in Flanders and Wallonia during the nineteenth century.

The process of secularisation (i.e. the gradual shift away from Roman Catholicism) was especially strong in Wallonia and penetrated deeply into remote villages. In Flanders, adherence to organised religion remained much more intact. At the turn of the century, only the large urban centres in the North were affected by secularisation. Its extent may be revealed, for example, through the amount of votes for non-Catholic parties. When the elections were first held on the basis of one man, one vote (1919) such differences were distinct. The Walloon industrial belt easily reached sixty or more percent of non-Catholic voters, whereas the arrondissements in the Ardennes had a smaller proportion of non-Catholic votes (rarely exceeding 50%). In contrast, the proportion of the non-Catholic vote in the more rural Flanders was nearly always below 40%. Exceptions to this regional trend were found in the urban areas of Antwerp, Brussels, Ghent and Ostend.

In order to look at historical developments in the fertility-regulating pattern of the Belgian population we have to look at changes in fertility and nuptiality trends. These have been substantially documented for the period between 1800 and 1970 and for the period after World War II (1). Empirical data on the contraceptive behaviour of the (married) population only became available from 1966 onwards.

From the data on marital fertility, it may be inferred

that contraceptive practice became increasingly widespread following the 1860s in some parts of (industrialised) Wallonia. Gradually thereafter, contraceptive practice must have been adopted extensively in the rest of Wallonia, in the Flemish urban areas, and finally in the Flemish countryside. What sort of methods were used to achieve this unprecedented degree of fertility control? Although undoubtedly abortion was practised, nobody has any idea about its incidence at that time. Abstinence and withdrawal were the major methods of fertility control. As late as 1966, the first national fertility survey discovered that nearly 41% of married couples were still practicing coitus interruptus. Clear regional differences were still noted at that time. Fertility control measures were probably adopted by the population at the cost of well-being in sexual life.

Why this conservatism with regard to contraceptive use? It is possible to consider the following factors in this respect (2):

- Catholic church hostility to fertility control;
- nationalistic reaction to the human slaughter of World War I;
- fear by Walloon socialists of demographic decline in their region (i.e. their electorate), in comparison with a predominantly Catholic dominated Flanders;
- lack of neo-Malthusian pressure groups within or outside the political party structure.

It may be said that the Catholic Church in Belgium, which maintained a strong moral authority, took the lead at that time in the western European drive against contraception. It initially voiced strong opposition to the notion of family limitation in general. Unlike France, Belgium took only a few decades to reduce marital fertility to unprecedentedly low levels in nearly all regions of the country.

The Church was facing a rapid spread of both 'onanism' (coitus interruptus) and secularisation at the same time. Well known is the letter of the Primate of Belgium in 1909 (Mercier), 'About the duties of married life' containing specific guidelines for the parish clergy. This reaction could only slow down the spread of contraceptive practice among more faithful Catholics as the control of fertility was already in an advanced stage especially in Wallonia.

The position of the Workers' Party towards fertility regulation was also quite unfavourable. To some extent the classic Marxist view was held: a declining population will adversely affect the growth of the Socialist-voting lower classes. In addition, the fact that population growth was considerably higher in predominantly Catholic Flanders than in predominantly Socialist Wallonia was not viewed with enthusiasm. The defenders of contraception remained very few and did not belong to the party elite.

Unlike England or the Netherlands, the neo-Malthusian pressure groups hardly had a chance to grow into a fully developed movement. In 1912, the 'Belgian league for the regulation of family size' was created. It remained a small set of inspired and motivated individuals boycotted by Catholics, liberals and socialists alike. They moved into Flanders from across the Dutch border and emerged in a few circles in Wallonia. World War I put an end to their activities. A family planning organisation would re-emerge only in 1955.

In summary, the spread of contraception in Belgium can be described as a silent process. The matter was hardly discussed publicly, let alone in a positive way, at least until the seventies. A general climate of shame prevailed. In spite of the availability of modern contraceptive methods, almost the entire population still appeared to have had sufficient motivation to resort to the sexually less satisfying forms of contraception and to the practice of abortion.

Substantial changes occurred in Belgian society after World War II. In 1948, women were given the vote (which men had had since 1919). In spite of substantial socio-economic development, the fifties were characterised by two major political and social problems: the attitude adopted by King Leopold III during World War II and the battle for the school system. The former was resolved by the succession to the throne in 1952 of his son, the latter by a complex School Treaty in 1958. Both problems revealed strong ideological and sub-regional (linguistic) differences which persisted after the conflict was formally resolved. Besides, a substantial (socio-economic) shift took place in Belgium. Flanders witnessed a process of rapid industrialisation initially in the areas of Antwerp and Ghent. New plants were introduced: motor industry, oil refinery, and chemical industries. Comparatively, Wallonia was left with older types of industries and infrastructure as well as an ageing population. As a result, the economic and banking power did not remain so exlusively in the Francophone part of the country. Moreover, Flanders held an increasing proportion of the Belgian population. This resulted in a revival of the longstanding demands of the Flemish-speaking part of the population. It reached the level of a broad political confrontation, leading to the first important change in the Constitution in 1970, introducing regional and cultural autonomy.

The 'Golden Sixties' in Belgium gave way to the so-called communautarian problems of the seventies, resulting in a second change in the Belgian Constitution in 1980, delegating responsibilities and some power to the Flemish and the Francophone communities. Cultural issues and matters affecting the individual (e.g. health, welfare) became matters to be decided at the level of the community rather than at the national level.

Legislation relating to planned parenthood:

General considerations

The Belgian legal attitude to the sexual behaviour of the population (3) may indeed be characterised as conservative, coercive, marriage-centred, and linking sexuality to procreation, as reflected in the in the Civil and Penal Codes.

The Civil Code is largely based on the 19th century Code Napoleon. For example it proclaims the primacy of marriage (i.e. discrimination against consensual unions), divorce as a punishment, the absolute power of parents over children, and discrimination against children born illegitimately.

Fundamental principles of the Belgian legislative system such as equality and personal freedom are quite frequently disregarded when it comes to sexuality and family life. Expressions of human sexuality, other than (marital) heterosexuality, are looked upon as indecent and are combatted. Belgian legislation in this domain has already been ruled in opposition to international legislation (e.g. the European Convention on Human Rights) in the case of the status of the child (1979) and of transsexuality (1980).

The Social Security and Fiscal Codes also affect

family life, the former not discriminating against the legal status of the child. Important changes occurred over the last two decades, concerning inheritance, the status of spouses, divorce and legislation affecting children.

Family planning services

Family planning services are provided mainly through the general health system via GPs and gynaecologists in private practice and/or clinics. It is fair to say that the government also involved itself indirectly by recognising and subsidising counselling centres dealing in part with family planning. Such recognition was accorded by an Act of 3 April, 1970 (BS/MB 17.4.70) for the 'Centres for pre-marital, marital, and family counselling'. Such centres had to 'provide the means to prepare youth for marital and parental status, to make parents aware of their duties towards their children, and to inform marriage partners on family planning'.

The timing of this regulation is largely attributed to the presence in the cabinet of the socialist Minister of Public Health - a well-known family planning volunteer. It included both bureaux for marriage and family counselling (more Catholic-inspired services) and family planning centres (more liberal/atheistic-inspired services), both of which emerged as a result of private initiatives during the 1960s.

By an Act of 11 March 1974 (MB/BS 19.4.74), the tasks of these centres were modified in order 'to provide at least one of the following services: information on family planning and contraceptives, and provision of contraceptives on request; guidance of family members experiencing relationship problems; practical assistance to women with unwanted pregnancies'.

This change may be looked at as making family planning more available through such services. However, the clause 'at least one of' resulted in a number of centres refusing to offer family planning (especially in Flanders). Moreover, the Ministry of Public Health did not mention in its brochure on contraception for the public (1974) the names and addresses of the centres it subsidised.

At the time of the regionalisation of Belgium, this domain became 'matters affecting the individual' no longer to be ruled on at the national level. However, only the Brussels region reformulated (in 1978) the aim of such centres more in accordance with the original aims. It was able as well to provide a more advantageous financial status for these counselling centres in comparison with Flanders and Wallonia.

After the change in the Belgian Constitution in 1980, this matter was subsumed within the jurisdiction of the communities. The Francophone Community accordingly developed a different regulation for "Centres d'aide et d'information sexuelle, conjugale et familiale" (Act of 22 December 1983 - MB/BS 3.2.84). It stipulates the following tasks:

- intake, information, and guidance in order to help people solve their sexual and relationship problems, as well as to help them in their educational task in this area;
- providing information on fertility regulation and offering the appropriate contraceptives on request;
- providing the basic notions of family legislation;
- providing education and information for adults and adolescents in the domain of sexual, emotional and relational life and of responsible parenthood;
- practical assistance to women with unwanted pregnancies.

The Flemish Community still acts according to the regulation of 1976. However, the Minister of the Family and Welfare Care commissioned in 1983 an advisory ruling on these centres from the High Council of the Family. The advice may be interpreted as not giving a high profile to family planning services via such counselling centres. Besides, according to the majority point of view such centres would also not be involved in preventive activities (information and education). A new regulation is expected by the end of 1984.

Contraceptives

By Act of 9 July 1973 (MB/BS 9.8.73) the paragraphs of Article 383 in the Penal Code prohibiting the publicity for and the distribution of contraceptives were abolished. Contraceptives were labelled and dealt with as 'medicaments', exception being made for the condom and the diaphragm. It accordingly required their registration, placed restrictions on some types of publicity, and necessitated a prescription. At first, the above-mentioned centres were allowed (if asking for a licence) to stock and distribute contraceptives. The State Council ruled this particular Act out of order in 1975, after the League of Doctors and League of Pharmacists made objections. Oral contraceptives were reimbursed through the Social Security system until 1980. The first bill proposing to change the prohibitive and ambigious law of 1923 was introduced in February 1966. Several others followed in vain. This sudden change in Belgian legislation on contraception is generally understood as an attempt to moderate public preoccupation with the abortion issue. As such, contraception was not regarded by some of the most influential decision-makers of that time as being of intrinsic value, but as instrumental in preventing a change in abortion legislation.

Within the context of an information campaign on responsible parenthood, an Act of 11 January 1974 (BS/MB 1.2.74, subsequently changed in 1974, 1976, 1977) made financial provision for courses or information sessions on contraception. Recognised organisations dealing with family educational activities and centres for family counselling are empowered to organise either training courses or general information sessions for adults or adolescents. No detailed statistics or analyses are available on the subsidising of such activities. Some figures were released (1973-76) through a brochure of the Minister of Public Health presenting the results of his campaign. Some information is available through the annual reports of the administration implementing this decree (4). Subject to quite specific conditions, subsidies were also given for publications on contraception, if made available to the membership through the journal of an organisation. To this end, the government has spent at most, half a million Belgian francs annually in Flanders, whereas approximately one and a half million was spent in Wallonia.

It is also interesting to take into account the rules concerning the subsidising of family life education activities.

Availability/sale of family planning related literature

Strictly speaking, no legal impediments exist to the availability and/or sale of family planning related literature. However, information can be judged pornographic and as such contrary to 'good morals' according to Article 383 of the Penal Code. Additionally, a law of 1936 allows the Belgian government to prohibit the import of foreign obscene publications.

It happened on several occasions that issues of a periodical or publications which the (Flemish) family planning centres distributed to their membership were recalled or at least withheld, either by the customs or by post office. Having no censorship in sensu strictu, such matters are ruled on at the local level. Before the Act of 1973 the diffusion of information on family planning was substantially limited and had a clandestine aura.

Since 1973, there has been a boom in publications dealing with contraception. Leaflets, brochures, or series of articles have been published by organisations with a rather wide membership (e.g. Family Movement Association and two major women's organisations), by pharmaceutical concerns, by consumer organisations, by a youth organisation, etc. They moved into the domain occupied by the family planning association in previous decades, albeit with much more modest means.

In addition, in 1974 the Ministry of Public Health published 900,000 copies of a brochure 'Contraception and Responsible Parenthood' in three languages. Separately, a booklet with more detailed information was distributed to doctors, pharmacists, midwifes, nurses, and certain categories of social workers.

This printed material, mainly directed at (married) adults, was restricted to details of reproduction. Rather than putting contraceptive information within the perspective of a view on human sexuality and social life, it was kept technical in order to satisfy a delusion, especially held by the authorities, of remaining ideologically neutral.

In 1982, the Ministry of the Francophone Community took responsibility for a brochure, initially from the city of Liège, and distributed 70,000 copies. It differs from the brochure distributed at the national level in at least two respects: the information is again more strictly medical, while however mentioning the addresses of centres subsidised by the government offering information on family planning. Specific reference is made to those providing medical consultation. A third edition (1984) is in press. In 1983, the Ministry of the Flemish Community edited a slightly updated version of the brochure, previously distributed by the Ministry of Public Health (1977 version). No mention is made of addresses of counselling centres providing family planning information and services.

Sterilisation

There is no law in Belgium covering sterilisation <u>per se</u>. As a surgical intervention, it comes under the heading of the Penal Code, stipulating penalties for deliberately inflicting wounds on another if not all conditions are met for a medical treatment:

- consent of the patient, with certain exceptions;
- adequate information on the nature of possible risks and the consequences of the intervention;
- to be a 'treatment';
- prognostication of success/failure ratio.

The law regarded sterilisation as a permissible method of contraception only if other reversible methods could not be used. This hampered the availability of sterilisation on contraceptive grounds. During the sixties and even part of the seventies, in quite a number of gynaecological centres an arbitrary set of conditions was put into practice: being married, being 30-35+ years old and having two or three children. Vasectomy was seldom considered. The more recent developments in the incidence of female and male sterilisation hint at substantial changes having occurred over the last five years.

Abortion

According to the Belgian Penal Code of 1867 the practice of abortion is severely punishable on any grounds.
Reference to this is found in the Penal Code, Book II, Title VII, 'of crimes and offences against the order of the family and against public decency', of which chapter 1 is entitled 'Abortion'. It includes Articles 348 to 353, which ban abortion without exception. Both the voluntary performer and the consenting woman are punishable by two to five years of imprisonment, plus a fine. Lesser punishments are applied if the abortion was accidentally induced through battery, if the abortion fails, or if extenuating circumstances can be cited. More severe charges are brought against the performer if the woman did not consent, if she dies, or if the abortionist belongs to

the (para) medical profession. An additional provision is to be found in chapter 7 ('public offence of good morals') of the same title. Article 383, introduced in 1923, pertains to abortion, pornography, and until 1973, contraception. It forbids all publicity, information and help regarding abortion.

It is within the discretionary powers of the Public Prosecutor to prosecute or not in certain cases. Whereas clandestine abortion has almost always been prosecuted (to the extent it could be proven), it is a longstanding tradition in Belgium not to prosecute in the case of abortion performed to save the woman's life. In general, the actual number of prosecutions and sentences is obviously far below the estimated number of performed abortions.

From 1968 to 1972, for example, 169 performers of abortion, and 132 women who had had abortions were convicted.

Due to the separation of powers, the Minister of Justice cannot, in principle, direct the practice of the Judiciary. It is known however that he may 'de facto' use his influence to suspend prosecutions. This influence was brought into play during the seventies as the politicians 'planned' to reform the abortion law.

Legislative initiatives related to abortion

Since 1971, about twenty bills were introduced, mainly from MPs of the socialist or of the liberal party. Most were never debated in Parliament mainly due to political instability. As Parliament disbands whenever the government falls, all bills have to be re-introduced. At present, two motions first tabled in 1978 still await discussion: one emanating from liberal MPs proposes to liberalise abortion while retaining some conditions; a bill stemming from socialist MPs aims at legalising abortion on request without imposing examination panels or delays between first consultation and the interruption of pregnancy.

Additionally, several proposals for the temporary suspension of the penal law on abortion have been forwarded. At first such bills were regarded as unconstitutional as they implied suspension of prosecution. In 1982, while several cases were pending before the criminal court in Brussels, such a proposal failed by only three votes (5).

Government involvement and initiatives

In the first half of 1972, the Minister of Justice consulted representatives of numerous organisations, university departments, and pressure groups on the abortion issue. This report showed clearly a number of points of agreement and disagreement (6).

By an Act of 13 December 1974 (BS/MB 17.12.74) a State Commission for the Study of Ethical Problems was established in order to provide the government with 'scientifically based advice on the issues of contraception, abortion, and the anonymity of the mother and of the child born in anonymity'. Twenty-five members were appointed by the government, selected according to criteria of language, politics, profession, religion and sex. Discord revealed itself most clearly on the abortion issue. In May 1976 the Commission advised some kind of depenalisation of abortion. Shortly afterwards, the minority vote-members (twelve) submitted a separate report defending the application of the existing law, with exceptions made only for medically-indicated abortions.

Since 1977, through policy declarations, successive governments have left the initiative to parliamentarians, considering that the abortion issue posed too great a threat of political disruption. The kind of strategies used by government to remain in control of the abortion issue are described below.

Infertility treatment

Whereas procreation is thoroughly dealt with by Belgian legislation, the biological inability to procreate is not taken care of other than through adoption. It was previously noted that the link between sexuality and procreation remains explicit in the Civil and Penal Code. As such, it is basically unsuitable for those situations where neither is involved. For example, artificial donor-insemination or in-vitro fertilisation are not yet dealt with. The practice of the former is dealt with nowadays by the courts, albeit hesitatingly in some cases. One definitely needs the consent of the woman, the husband, and the donor. Absolute secrecy is required. Article 88 of the Code of Medical Ethics deals with this item. The status of the child born from donor insemination remains an important problem. A draft resolution of the Committee of Ministers of the Council of Europe (1979) has probably stimulated thinking at the level of Belgian legislation. In 1982, a Bill was introduced within the Council of the Francophone Community relating to artificial donor-insemination.

Sex/family life education

This subject is not included in the school curriculum by governmental provision.

This non-inclusion can be related to the value-based character of such instruction, and to the division of the Belgian school system, mainly based on a denominational segregation ('verzuiling'/'cloisonnement'). There are the 'official' (state/neutral) and the 'free' (Catholic) schools. The former are under the direct supervision of the Minister of Education, the latter are ruled by an independent national Board. Both are subsidised by the State.

In general, much depends on the attitude taken by the local Board, and of the teachers who could possibly deal with aspects of sex/family life education. Although no survey evidence is available on the subject, it is likely that such education became more widespread during the seventies. Within the State school system, a general item 'sexual and emotional guidance' is introduced in the general programme directory at the level of the secondary schools. Within the free school system, a number of more specific instructions govern the conduct of the teachers.

A Bill relating to sex/family life education, was first introduced at the level of the Council of the Francophone Community in 1980, aimed to cover emotional, familial, and sexual education at the different levels of the school system. Another followed in 1982, resulting after a number of amendments in a Decree of 10 July 1984 (MB/BS 22.8.84) of the Executive of the Communauté Française relating 'a l'education sanitaire et l'information de la jeunesse ainsi qu'a l'aide et a l'assistance aux familles, dans les domaines rélatifs à la contraception et à la parente résponsable'.

Article 4 stipulates that schools in the Francophone community have to organise, in coordination with the counselling (family planning) centres, information dealing with the juridical, technical, moral and medical aspects of parenthood and contraception. The minister in charge submitted an amendment, suggesting that such information be given within the framework of courses of biology, social sciences, or ethics.

One may also take into account the rules providing for subsidies for activities promoting family education, the development of family life, and the training of persons in charge of family formation courses (for adults). These subsidies were provided for by a 1978 Act (modifying previous ones of 1949, 1959 and 1974). These activities have to deal with marital life, the interrelationships between family members, the sexual and emotional education, family education, hygiene, childcare, domestic management, and domestic chores.

In previous years the administrative application forms had provided contraception be included in the above. However, these subsidies have been taken up in a remarkably uneven way between Dutch-speaking and French-speaking organisations (approx. 80/20). During the early 1980s, about 38 million Belgian francs were provided to the former for such family-oriented activities. The use of these funds increased substantially following the Act of 1978 as it doubled the subsidy for such courses. No similar substantial increase was ever provided for information sessions on contraception.

Adoption

Legislation on adoption rapidly evolved during the 20th century in Belgium. At present, a 1969 Act (MB/BS 12.4.69) governs the practice of adoption. Compared to previous laws of 1940, 1951 and 1958, it is more child-oriented. A change in legislation on adoption was discussed by the State Commission for the Study of Ethical Problems. In addition, a proposal of law (1978) relating to the status of the child includes some implications for adoption. As yet, it has not been dealt with.

Two types of adoption exist: ordinary adoption and legitimation through adoption. The latter gives the adoptee the same rights as the legal child of the adoptees, and breaks all previous links with the biological parent/s. It accounts for about three quarters of all adoptions occuring in Belgium (approx 4,000 annually) (7).

Adopters should be married couples with at least one

of the spouses is thirty years old, if the marriage is less than five years' duration. If a parent wants to adopt its 'natural' child or if the adoption relates to a child of one of the spouses, it suffices that the adopter is 21 and ten years older than the adoptee.

The procedural requirements are complex, aiming to be of most advantage to the child.

Country situation: quantitative data

This section aims to document (statistically) the planned parenthood situation in the country. Use will be made of data available through census, surveys, opinion polls, etc. relating to the fertility and the fertility regulating behaviour of the population. The focus is on recent developments and trends (mainly after World War II). (5-6)

Demographic situation

Belgium had a population of 9,853,023 inhabitants in 1983. The rate of growth is marginally above zero (0.1% in 1981-82). In the 20th century longevity doubled as elsewhere in Western Europe. While the demographic situation in Belgium is apparently static, there is a difference in movement between the regions and communities in the country (Table 1).

Table 1: Demographic development in Belgium of the different linguistic regions.

REGIONS	1961	1970	1980	1982
Dutch-speaking	55.1	56.1	57.2	57.4
French-speaking	33.2	32.1	32.0	31.9
German-speaking	0.6	0.7	0.7	0.7
Brussels	11.1	11.1	10.1	10.0
n=100%	9,189,741	9,605,944	9,848,647	9,858,017

Source: Belgian report to International Conference on Population, 1984, p. 3

The Flemish population rose as a result of natural

increase and of migration. The population of the bilingual region Brussels-capital declined as a result of a natural decrease and movement out of the city, both factors having a negative effect. The population of Wallonia increased (in absolute numbers) only because of migration into the region, the natural demographic development being negative. The small population of the German-speaking region maintained its same relative proportion as a result of a continuing increase.

In a situation where migration has such a role to play, the foreign population of Belgium has more than quadrupled in the 20th century. Foreigners numbered little more than 200,000 in 1900; they now number more than 900,000. The numbers of the foreign population vary considerably from one region to another: in 1981 15% of the foreign population resided in Wallonia, 31% in Brussels and 4% in Flanders.

As with some other European countries, Belgium witnessed a decline in fertility from 1964. At that time, there were approximately 161,000 births per annum. This drop continued until 1975, after which a modest increase was noted, being the result of a favourable age structure (more women between 20-29 years old) and a levelling out of fertility rates. This age structure effect will continue to be favourable until the early nineties.

Table 2: Total fertility in Belgium (1950-1980)

1950 : 2.34	1970 : 2.25
1955 : 2.38	1975 : 1.73
1960 : 2.54	1980 : 1.69
1965 : 2.61	

Source: Willems et al., 1981, p. 286 (8).

This fall was apparent in every region, leading in 1982 to a birthrate which was the same everywhere. Consequently, the regional differences in natural growth are the result of a higher death rate in the regions with an older population (Wallonia and Brussels), and of a lower death rate in the regions with a less aged population (Flanders and the German-speaking region). In general, the increase in the foreign population disguises the recent, real reduction in the population of Belgian nationality.

Case Study: Belgium

Nuptiality/divorce

Births occur mainly within marriage in Belgium. The rate of out of wedlock births was less than 3% in the period 1950-1975, rising to 4.5% in 1981.

During the decade 1970-1980 important changes occurred in the field of nuptiality. Whereas 98 first marriages took place per 100 women in 1970, only 74 were observed in 1981 (cross-sectional sum of age-specific first marriage rates). This is a decline of 24%. In comparison with other Western European countries, the propensity to marry remains relatively high in Belgium and even more so in Flanders. This rapid decline is brought about by the interaction of two phenomena: postponement of marriage and non-marriage. Up to now, most signs point towards unwillingness: the first marriage rates at older ages remain fixed at a low level instead of increasing. Furthermore, one notes decreasing remarriage by divorced women and widows.

From 1970 to 1981, the duration-specific divorce rates more than doubled at each duration of marriage. It is expected that more than 25% of marriages will be dissolved after a duration of twenty years, in the marriage cohorts that started after 1975.

Contraceptive use

Empirical evidence on the contraceptive use of the Belgian population is available from 1966. For the Flemish community, data are available, mainly for women aged 20-45 years old, for 1975-76 and 1982-83. For the Francophone community, the latest data on contraceptive use were collected in the second half of the seventies.

During the sixties and the early seventies, it was noted that the married population in the Francophone part of the country made use of more effective, 'modern' methods of contraception, compared to Flanders. This was largely influenced by the behavioural pattern in the Brussels region. Only data are presented for the married population in Flanders (see Table 3). On the basis of comparable empirical data until the mid-seventies, it may be supposed that such data most probably hold as well for the rest of the country.

The development in the contraceptive use over a period of fifteen years may be characterised as a 'contraceptive revolution'. Interestingly, the use of mechanical contraceptives (condom, diaphragm) remained low during those years.

Table 3: The contraceptive use of 20-24 year olds and of 40-44 year-old married women in Flanders, 1966 and 1983.

Age	20-24		40-44	
Year:	1966	1983	1966	1983
Use:	56	67	79	89
Non use:	44	33	21	11
Method				
Coitus Interruptus (CI)	60	8	56	13
Periodic Abstinence (PA)	18	2	24	8
CI and PA.	3	5	4	10
Douche	1	–	7	–
Condom/Diaphragm	8	7	4	8
IUD	–	7	–	5
Orals	10	70	4	18
Sterilisation	1	1	1	37

Source: Population and Family Study Centre, National Fertility Surveys, 1966 and 1982-83.

Abortion

By the end of the seventies, domestic abortion declined, with Belgian women going to the Netherlands or the UK. By 1981, an analysis became available on the basis of information from outpatient clinics in the Netherlands (STIMEZO, Permanent Registration) and through data collated in the French-speaking part of Belgium by GACEHPA (Action group of outpatient clinics performing abortion). Both sets of data relate to 1979.

Abortion facilities are mainly developed in the French-speaking part of the country. Except for a number of extra-hospital centres performing pregnancy terminations on request, there are a few hospitals considering treatments on grounds wider than strictly medical indications. Altogether they treated more than 7,000 (mainly French-speaking) women for abortion.

Additionally, some 8,000 to 8,500 (mainly Dutch-speaking) women annually travel to abortion centres in the Netherlands. If these figures are complete, there would be about one induced abortion for each nine to ten births in Belgium.

Thus, in spite of the repressive legislation in Belgium at least 15,000 Belgian women seek an abortion in or outside the country annually. Access to abortion facilities differs for Dutch-speaking and French-speaking women. The former need to travel mainly either to the Netherlands or to the southern part of Belgium, whereas the latter are mainly helped within or nearby their place of residence.

Belgium is divided on the subject of abortion. Yet, since 1972, a clear-cut evolution in public opinion is to be noted, increasingly favouring a less rigorous application of the law. This opinion was expressed, among others, in the context of the European Value Systems Study (1981). In general, a large majority of the population is in favour of abortion relating to specific indications (woman's life being endangered, risk of malformed child); a minority favour it in the case of more general conditions (e.g. unmarried woman, married couple not wanting children). Differences remain on the basis of linguistic or ideological characteristics of the respondents.

An inquiry conducted among politicians in 1978 (project European Parties' Middle Level Elites of the European Elections Study) showed that no political party was homogeneous regarding this matter. The majority of the Members of Parliament stated that they personally favoured depenalisation. The difference between personal opinion and vote in Parliament may be explained by the imperatives of party coherence and the desire to avoid a government crisis. Most recently, for example, a number of liberal MPs who had previously claimed to be in favour of new legislation voted along with their Catholic coalition partners against the proposal for temporary suspension of the law.

Infertility treatment

No overall data are available on the number of artificial donor inseminations or other interventions performed to increase fertility.

In general, it was estimated recently on the basis of the results of the Fertility Survey that 3% of the married female population has to cope with primary sterility and 6% with secondary sterility (sub-fertility).

Adoption

As can be noted from Table 4, the number of adoptions increased steadily in Belgium in previous decades. This increase was most pronounced after changes in legislation in 1958 and 1969.

Table 4: Number of adoptions in Belgium, 1950-1980

1950 :	814	1970 :	2,553	1980 :	4,048
1960 :	1,256	1975 :	2,893		

Source: *Statistical Yearbook of Belgium*, 1982, Volume 102, p. 70.

However, such an increase hides the problem of abandoned children in Belgium. As a matter of fact, the largest number of adoptions are formalities for legal purposes. An increasing amount of hetero-familial adoptions is to the benefit of non-Belgian children. Handicapped children are seldom adopted.

COUNTRY SITUATION: QUALITATIVE DATA

Compared with other issues, planned parenthood in Belgium has received meagre attention. It is felt that a number of characteristics within Belgian society may explain this.

The meaning of planned parenthood

Planned parenthood has ideological significance beyond the term 'fertility regulation'.

There are three interconnected areas of conflict in Belgian society: the ideological (Roman Catholic/atheist), the linguistic (Flemish/Walloon), and the socio-economic (employees/employers).

The strong opposition of the Roman Catholic hierarchy

Roman Catholicism is the predominant religion, with a major difference between the north and south. The north (Flanders) remains more Catholic than the south (Wallonia). At the beginning of the 20th century, family limitation was strongly combatted (see Section 2). During the sixties and much of the seventies, the use of 'artificial' contraceptives was still opposed. Nowadays, only the Bishop of Ghent remains the spokesman for the most traditional point of view on contraceptive use. Since the early seventies, attention mainly focussed on the abortion issue.

In the 1980s Roman Catholicism has declined in popularity and it is unclear to what extent this may influence the position taken by the Church authorities on planned parenthood.

The attitude of the medical profession

It is obvious that the medical profession plays a crucial role in this area. A peculiarity of Belgian society makes this even more relevant. Through the League of Doctors (obligatory membership for every practising doctor), the medical profession is more or less autonomous. Belgium has no National Health service, therefore government has little control over private medical practice.

The 1923 law did not forbid the spread of scientific information on contraceptives. Nevertheless, it was not until the early sixties that student doctors received contraceptive information and training. Due to the characteristics of the medical school system in Belgium the impact of the authorities on the curriculum is limited, especially with regard to the training of doctors. As such, much still depends on the views of the persons in charge.

It is important to note the influence of the pharmaceutical industry which was responsible for bringing the oral contraceptive to the attention of physicians through marketing publicity for profit. It also organised seminars for the Belgian Family Planning Association.

The advent of oral contraception simultaneously stimulated and inhibited contraceptive training for doctors. The advantage of the pill from the doctors' point of view is that it may be prescribed without the technical knowledge required for diaphragm or the IUD insertion. The contraceptive choice of women has been seriously limited by the restricted knowledge and technical skills of a large part of the medical profession.

The non-involvement of important organisations

Some important organisations in the country, be it in terms of their membership, their geographical coverage, and/or their financial power, were not involved for many years in family planning despite the relationship of their activities to planned parenthood (e.g. the 'National Work for the Well-being of the Child' (ONE/NWK)). In spite of their contact with pregnant working class women they have not become involved in planned parenthood.

Only at the beginning of the seventies did the League of Large Families become involved. Being a pluralistic organisation it has had a strong Catholic influence at Board level. Although publication of a brochure on contraception in 1974 was a turning point, it was not so easy for the League to join the information campaign on contraception. For example, one of the most severe reactions came from an Honorary President - the Bishop of East Flanders - who denied the League the use of premises owned by the church. An organisation such as the League most probably helped to legitimise the use of contraceptives among couples traditionally not accustomed to such practice.

The major Catholic inspired women's organisation also became involved by discussing contraception and responsible parenthood with its membership in a series of articles (1973-74).

In contrast, the socialist-inspired women's organisation had always been more strongly involved. During the thirties, it campaigned for 'Conscious Motherhood' and the abolition of the paragraphs in the Penal Code concerning contraception. It is believed that their activity was restricted to some extent by its Francophone branch which was worried about the declining birthrate in Wallonia. During the sixties, the socialist women's organisation started a number of family planning services on their own (9) and now actively lobbies for the abolition of the prohibitive law on abortion.

The Family Planning Association: a modest pressure group

The family planning movement in the first decades of the 20th century had little public impact. After World War II another attempt was made to organise the advocates of planned parenthood in Belgium. In 1955, the 'Belgian League for Sexual Advice' was created. Again with the help from the family planning movement in the Netherlands (10).

Family planning services were first offered in Ghent (1960) and Antwerp (1961). By 1962, the first centre was opened in the Francophone part of the country ('La Famille Heureuse') followed by numerous other centres. Shortly afterwards a national family planning federation was created which joined the IPPF. It made a substantial contribution to the spread of the idea of family planning by organising a national symposium in 1970, successfully reaching several hundred doctors to inform them on contraceptive methods. A symposium on the 'Contraceptive Society' (1972) focused on the prohibitive legislation on contraception and abortion.

At the local level, many more family planning centres emerged in the Francophone part of the country, especially in the Brussels region. Only twenty five percent of the counselling centres subsidised by the government offer family planning services in Flanders compared with more than two thirds of such centres in the French-speaking part of Belgium.

The family planning movement in Belgium has never been solely concerned with contraceptives but also devotes itself to tackling taboos on sexuality and opposing puritanical ideas. This has been opposed by those linking family planning with an obsessive interest in sex.

There are other reasons for the isolation of the family planning movement in Belgium. Resistance to Roman Catholic attitudes to procreation from liberals and freemasons produced strong Catholic reaction.

At first, the majority of female volunteers were middle-class, even well-to-do people, providing information and help to those living in cities. However, during the seventies, younger people with feminist and academic backgrounds took over. They introduced political action (urging repeal of prohibitive practices and legislation) and introduced psycho-sexual counselling into family planning centres.

The small family planning movement has also been

fundraising, providing information and training for its volunteers, struggling with legal and administrative constraints, and creating new family planning services.

There is little solid data on the extent to which family planning centres are known to and used by the public. It is suspected that their impact is modest, with a selected clientele. Compared with other services their bias was previously towards the privileged, educated part of the population. Recently, the bias has been in favour of younger people, who are considered an important target group for such services.

The role of the authorities: reluctant and 'neutral

The involvement of Belgian authorities in planned parenthood affairs has stemmed from two concerns: the need to combat 'crimes and misbehaviour against the order of the family and public morals'; and fear over the slow but steady decline in the birthrate.

Both conform with the views of the Catholic Church relating to procreation and sexuality. An anecdote illustrates this conformity. In January 1965 an MP made a point in Parliament about the problems of family planning in Belgium. The Minister of Public Health and the Family replied there was no need to hurry as long as the Vatican Council had not yet announced its views on the matter!

Key departments involved in planned parenthood are the Ministry of Public Health (and the Family), and the Ministry of Justice. The former was most frequently ruled by a member of the Christian Democratic Party (CVP/PSC), guaranteeing control over legislation in this area.

As previously noted, it took the Belgian government until 1973 to abolish restrictions on contraceptives, when a subject which had been opposed for so many years was quite suddenly 'promoted' as important to healthy marital and family life. It is generally agreed that the <u>de facto</u> situation was given legal sanction in order to avoid a direct confrontation on the abortion issue.

Indeed, the Government was confronted in early 1973 with social turmoil after a well-known gynaecologist was jailed for announcing that he had performed several hundred abortions. The gap between the legal and factual situation became more glaring. In spite of legislative change on contraception rather than abortion, Catholic opposition remained. A powerful politician was needed to give status to this reform. He argued that the government information campaign was not contraceptive propaganda, but a campaign for responsible parenthood.

The Ministry of Public Health said 25 million francs would be spent on an information campaign on contraception, though it was never publicly documented how this was spent. Nevertheless, in 1977 the Ministry produced two brochures: 'Responsible Parenthood' and 'Intake Structures for the Family'.

The abortion issue was defused by the creation of a State Commission, the recommendations of which were ignored as they did not conform with conservative opinion. Increasingly short-lived governments have since become involved with community tensions and other changes in the Belgian Constitution. Thus there has been little time for creative policy-making in planned parenthood. At best, lip service has been paid to sex/family life education and to the importance of centres for marital counselling and family planning.

As planned parenthood issues more and more became the responsibility of the communities, the prospect of increased attention and sound policy-making emerged. It has been noted that this process was recently initiated.

IMPLICATIONS/RECOMMENDATIONS

Overall, it appears that the factual situation has resulted from a number of hidden and silent changes in the mentality and behaviour of the population. While many people publicly acquiesced to religious authority, they conducted their affairs according to their consciences.

Belgian authorities never developed an overall policy encouraging planned parenthood as a basic human right. Most of the influential groups and organisations in society certainly did not pressure them to do so. They rather presented themselves as defenders of public morals and tried to halt the decline of the birthrate. They prefer to present the image of remaining 'neutral' in these affairs.

Until now, no explicit population policy has been declared by the government. It claimed to be more concerned about a family policy. Such measures aim at improving the living conditions, the health and/or the well-being of families. In this respect, specific planned parenthood issues have been given a low profile.

To the extent that policy measures relate to the provision of family planning services outside of private medical practice, a number of administrative regulations and duties hamper rather than facilitate the process. No policy has until now been directed at children/adolescents to provide them with a sound and consistent preparation in human relations, sexuality and procreation.

The Government should consider:

1   Decriminalising certain planned parenthood issues (such as abortion);
2   Monitoring the availability of family planning methods and services;
3   Eliminating discrimination against children on the basis of the marital status of their parents;
4   Providing education for adolescents and adults alike relating to sex roles and family life;
5   Taking positive action on the adoption of deprived children;
6   Stimulating research into psycho-social aspects of methods of fertility regulation;
7   Monitoring the curriculum of the medical and para-medical professions with a view to including family planning training;
8   Counteracting inequalities in provision of sex/family life education, adoption and artificial insemination;
9   That the notion of the traditional family is a prescriptive or normative ideological concept which does not necessarily fit the social reality today;
10   The dangers of labelling social problems as family problems (e.g. those arising from housework, shift-work); as well as labelling family problems (e.g. unwanted pregnancy, divorce) as ethical problems.

On the subject of planned parenthood Belgium seems to be at a crossroads. At present, some of the issues are still dealt with at the national level (e.g. abortion, adoption), though others are now within the jurisdiction of the community, which offers new possibilities for social change.

REFERENCES:

1.   Lesthaeghe, R. The Decline of Belgian Fertility, 1800-1970 1977 Princeton University Press; 'A Century of Demographic and Cultural Change in Western Europe: an Exploration of Underlying Dimensions' in Population and Development Review 1983, 9,3; Willems, P. et al.,'De evolutie van de vruchtbaarheid in Belgie, 1950-80' in Bevolking & Gezin 1981, 3 pp. 257-292.; Willems, P. & Wijewickrema, S. 'De evolutie van de nuptialiteit van 1954 tot 1981' in Bevolking & Gezin 1984.

2.   Stengers, J. 'Les pratiques anticonceptionelles dans le marriage au XIXe siecles: problemes humains et attitudes religieuses' in Revue Belge de Philosophie et d'Histoire 1971, 49, pp. 403-481, 1119-1174; Van Praag, Ph. 'De opkomst van het nieuw-malthusianisme in Vlaanderen' in T. Soc. Geschied. 1977.

3.   Coene, M.(red), Statuut van het kind Brussel, Ced-Samson 1980; Pauwels, J.M. Recht inzake seksualitiet 1982 Leuven, Uitg. Acco. (2).

4.   Ministerie van Volksgezondheid en van het Gezin. Bewustouderschap. Bericht over informatieverspreiding. (Dutch version). Brussel, Dienst Pers & Voorlichting, April 1977. Ministerie van Volksgezondheid. Jaarverslagen.

5.   Marques-Pereira, B. L'interruption volontaire de grossesse: un processus de politisation I+II, 1981 Bruxelles, CRISP (CH nr 923 CH nr 930-931). Claeys, P-H. & N. Loeb-Mayer, Les partis devant le problème de l'avortement, 1982 Bruxelles, CRISP (CH nr 962). GACEHPA, La pratique de l'avortement en Belgique. Etude statistique commentee, 1981 Bruxelles, Octobre.

6.   Ministerie van Justitie. Enige beschouwingen over het abortusvraagstuk (Dutch version). 1972 Brussel.

7.   Berckmans, P. e.a., Adoptie. Een rechts-sociologische benadering. 1981 A'pen/ A'dam, De Sikkel/De Ned. Boekhandel. Van Look, M. Evolutie van het Belgisch adoptierecht. T Privaatrecht, 1970, (4), 345-418.

8.   Willems P., Wijewickrema S., Lesthaeghe R. 'De evolutie van de bruchtbaarheid in Belgi, 1950-1980', Bevolking & Gezin, 1981, 3, 257-292. Willems P. & Wijewickrema S. 'De evolutie van de nuptialitiet van 1954 tot 1981' Bevolking & Gezin, 1984, 3 (in druk).

9.   Dille-Lobe V. 'Korte geschiedenis van de gezinsplanning in Belgie', <u>Social Standpunten</u> 1966, 175-182.

10.   Coulon F. 'Les centres de planning familial en Belgique', <u>Cedif Info</u>, 1981, N° 6, 1-18.   Rifflet, M. 'Le controle des naissances en Belgique', <u>La Nouvelle Revue</u>, 1973, 29e annee, 1, 29-34.

The Legal and Factual Status of Planned Parenthood in France

Y Blanpied, M-F Coulet and C Gallard

Before the war of 1870 the French Government encouraged the French not to be prolific, because of the special nature of the population of France in Europe. The French had been practising fertility control (coitus interruptus, abortifacients, etc.) for fifty years.

The Neo-Malthusian struggles

Following the 1870 war the Neo-Malthusians, who wanted to give working-class women effective means of controlling their own fertility, came into conflict with Government authorities officially opposed to freedom of choice in motherhood. This opposition was supported by the Protestant and Catholic Churches' view that contraception was to be regarded as a sin, and by moralists who regarded information about contraception as pornography.

Repression in silence

There followed many years of confrontation between the supporters of freedom of choice in motherhood (feminists, trades unionists, workers) and those who favoured an increasing birthrate (champions of traditional morality). After the 1914-18 war the latter, concerned by the depletion of the population, forced women back into the role of childbearer through legislation. In a climate where there was no longer a popular movement in favour of the freedom to choose motherhood, it was easy to pass the laws of 1920 and 1923 which criminalised abortion and suppressed contraceptive information, classing it as incitement to abortion.

In spite of these laws and the very severe repression which took place (66 convictions between 1920 and 1923) women continued to have abortions in increasing numbers. In addition these laws helped greatly to increase social inequality - in fact the better-off women were able to obtain abortions and contraceptives in neighbouring countries (England, Netherlands, Switzerland etc.), whereas the working class women were isolated and had nowhere to turn.

New dimensions in sexual liberation: the emergence of birth control

An action was brought against a woman teacher (1927) by those opposed to freedom of choice in motherhood, because of a sex/pre-marital education programme which appeared in the 'bulletin of the feminist groups of lay teachers' produced by Neo-Malthusians, the feminist press, lay organisations associated with the Defence of Democracy, the Communist Party and anarchists. The resulting trial had the merit of bringing questions about sexuality into the open and was a pretext for some to take up the struggle for women's freedom of choice in motherhood once again.

Faced with the awakening of public opinion, the political parties were forced to take a definite stand against the 1920 law, but they did so in the name of freedom of thought and not as champions of a woman's right to control her fertility. The Socialist and Communist parties each proposed a bill withdrawing the ban on contraceptive publicity, without success, even when the Left came to power in 1936.

During this period the feminist movements concentrated chiefly on the struggle for civic equality for women, which came up against strong opposition in the Senate.

The Neo-Malthusians continued to defend a woman's right to free, voluntary motherhood but they were not the only group involved. People with different political persuasions also took up the cause. For example, some militant anarchists were to introduce female contraceptives into France secretly, perform abortions and were even charged in connection with a vasectomy case (1935, see **Legislation**).

The supporters of scientific birth control distinguished between procreation and sexuality. For the supporters of birth control, therefore, demands for responsible sexuality and motherhood were substituted by those for birth control and sexual freedom. The concept of 'family planning' was born. The couple and the child - and no longer just the woman - became entities whose well-being was to be sought through scientific progress.

The Catholic Church, whose influence was dominant in France, maintained its opposition to all these ideas in spite of the changing view of a very small number of believers who were beginning to suggest that pleasure between husband and wife was not a sin.

On the other hand, the Secretary General of the French Communist Party expressed his opposition to contraceptive freedom. By deliberately likening the theory of 'birth control' to that of the Neo-Malthusians, the French Communist Party determined its opposition to any liberalisation of contraception and sexual behaviour for many years.

There were exceptional actions, like those of the French doctor, Jean Dalsace, who opened a clinic in a Paris suburb in order to inform women about existing contraceptive methods and gave them supplies in spite of the repression. Nevertheless, the general oppressive situation for women had not changed much by 1939.

The cloistering of women

In 1939 French women still did not have the right to vote, and according to their legal status they were subordinate to their husbands. The Code of the Family (27 July 1939) instituted measures promoting motherhood, social measures 'beneficial' to all, and measures intended to intensify the repression of abortion within the law (Art. 317 of the Penal Code), particularly as regards doctors and midwives, who then refused to give any assistance to women who had had abortions and sent them to the hospital regardless of the physical and legal risks involved. It was a triumph for the 'ideology of the family'.

After the armistice of 1940 the Petain regime, with Nazi and Fascist ideologies in the background, used the Code of the Family (1939) to proclaim loud and long: 'Bringing children into the world is woman's only function, her body does not belong to her, it is only the repository of the unborn child; bringing up children, looking after the home, serving her husband, this is a woman's duty, this should be her ideal'. The regime idealised the woman as mother by creating the Fête des Méres (Mother's Day) and considered the family as sacred.

It was a long way from the burgeoning, liberating ideas of the turn of the century. The apologia of the maternal function, the suppression of abortion and contraception had a profound effect on the attitudes, habits and even the structure of French society.

A changing society: 1945-1955

An order of 21 April 1944 from the provisional Government in Algiers, assumed by De Gaulle on 25 August 1944, acknowledged women's rights. The 1946 Constitution proclaimed sexual equality in all spheres. In concrete terms this decade represented the shift from repression to the era of the consumer society, including expenditure on health.

Instituted by the Order of 4 October 1945, the social security system was a recognition of everyone's right to health.

At the same time there was a considerable population increase (which students of demography explain as a short-lived consequence of any armed conflict), a reduction in infant mortality, an exodus from the country to Paris and the other large provincial cities, and high foreign immigration. Foreign workers and new city-dwellers were not sufficient to keep the new factories going and industry called extensively on female labour. The 'housing crisis' which arose as a result of this situation was to continue for a good many years. Finding somewhere to live was long to be the chief preoccupation of young couples and families on low incomes.

From a political point of view the constitutional declaration of sexual equality did not bridge the gap between theory and reality. Discrimination was to continue for a long time, particularly within marriage, where the wife still remained partly inferior, needing her husband's permission to continue in employment, for example.

On the political as well as the economic and professional levels, women were subject to the fluctuating needs of society. Used when needed, rejected when superfluous.

The reformist 'feminist' measures or half-measures instituted at the time of the Liberation created a brief pause in the feminist movement's struggle, as they corrected the most blatant discrimination. Nonetheless, an overall analysis of the female condition was never undertaken and there was no real change in male/female relationships, even with increasing liberalisation of social mores.

The gap between talk about sexual equality and the reality would one day become the basis of the struggle for free abortion.

In 1949 Simone de Beauvoir introduced those elements of publicity and thought needed in order to create a new dimension for feminism. The publication of The Second Sex was a major event. Twenty_two thousand copies were sold during the first week, probably because of the scandal caused by her relentless denunciation of the oppression suffered by women. Simone de Beauvoir's assessment was that of a pioneer and her views were misundertood and often distorted at first. In her account of sexual oppression she gives pride of place to the dramatic stories of confinements and illicit abortion (abortion was still severely repressed; in 1946 there were 5,251 prosecutions).

In the following decades, both in France and the USA, The Second Sex introduced to feminism generations of women who were increasingly to discover the meaning of its famous claim: 'one is not born a woman, one becomes one'. This view was to be the starting point and the point of reference for the various branches within the women's liberation movements. But French society was not ready to question the traditional roles of men and women, particularly within the family.

Maternity measures were introduced: family allowance, maternity grant, various grants relating to housing, education, tax reductions according to the number of children and, in parallel, taxes on the childless unmarried, widowed and divorced. In this changing society the immutable doctrine of the Catholic Church helped to restrain attitudes towards sexuality: 'The primary and intimate purpose of marriage is to bring forth and bring up new life.'

These attitudes, re-affirmed at all levels by the Catholic Church, explain why, in 1950, French couples did not always have effective contraceptives (apart from condoms, tolerated as protection against venereal disease). The Church tolerated natural methods only. The 1920 law remained in force, contributing towards sexual oppression of women because of the burden of the prohibitions and the fear of unwanted pregnancies.

The silence broken

During a visit to a birth control clinic in New York

Dr Marie-Andrée Weill Halle had been shocked by the work of family planning doctors which enabled women to avoid pregnancy. Years spent in medical practice and her experience of many dramatic cases were however gradually to lead her to share the view of her American colleagues. 'Encouraging the birth of children which a couple are able to bring up, helping couples to understand about organising their family harmoniously, helping parents to have wanted children - in this sense birth control is certainly a way of combatting abortion.' These 'shocking techniques' were without a doubt a 'lesser evil'.

In view of this development it seemed essential to her that these techniques should be made known. Thousands of couples would certainly be in favour of birth control, but it was a matter of being able to reach them, tell them about it. In Marie-Andrée Weill Halle's view this job was the doctor's, being in daily contact with people and families in their most intimate moments. She was to make several attempts, all vain, to interest the medical profession in birth control.

Different movements were thus converging towards the same objective: young Protestant women, freemasons, rationalists, Zionists, liberals and progressives and teachers all wanted to fight for wanted pregnancy.

An association 'La Maternité Heureuse' (Happy Motherhood) was founded in 1956 under the auspices of Lagroua-Weill-Halle. The choice of this name was motivated by the desire to obtain the support of a broad spectrum of people while responding to the founders' profound desire to relate essentially to women.

The rise of the MFPF

'La Maternité Heureuse' affiliated to the IPPF in 1958 and became the Mouvement Français pour le Planning Familial (French Family Planning Movement MFPF) in 1960. The association soon met weighty opposition from the Communist Party and the Catholic Church.

The French Communist Party, continuing to equate Neo-Malthusians and birth control, seized every opportunity to attack the supporters of responsible parenthood and also demonstrated the Stalinist puritanism which was so firmly entrenched in it at that time.

For its part the Catholic Church was scandalised to see the establishment of an association whose declared aim was to dissociate procreation from the sexual act. This continued to cause opposition between clerics and lay people, and the supporters of a secular Republic were to find themselves in the MFPF on the side of responsible parenthood. On the legislative front, several bills on birth control were put forward by various Leftist groups but came up against the inertia of political power.

La Maternité Heureuse organised itself against this opposition and held meetings to try to make the largely ignorant public and doctors aware of birth control.

Throughout these five years, the debate on contraception, restricted to an aware group of intellectuals and doctors, did not reach the public at large. There was therefore no reason for the politicians to take serious notice of these demands, and the traditional opponents of all liberalisation had no need to organise themselves in order to combat a handful of supporters.

The situation was to change radically when, thanks to the courageous initiative of convinced militants, the first MFPF information centres opened, in Grenoble in June 1961 and in Paris in the autumn, and were soon followed by many more. These centres, which were soon to offer the public both information and the possibility of a prescription and the supply of contraceptives, brought the MFPF from theoretical ideas to practical achievement. From the moment when 16,000 women were using contraceptives (the number of MFPF clients in January 1963) the period of secrecy was over, the silence was broken, the MFPF had created a fait accompli. The rapid expansion of the Movement, the crowds at its centres, its presence throughout the country, were to help to prove that there was a real need for contraception in the population, a need hypocritically hidden for more than forty years by draconian legislation effectively reinforced by rigorous repression.

The family planning activists did so well in spreading contraception that in 1965 the politicians found themselves forced to consider the matter publicly:

-   a motion on the subject was submitted to the National Socialist Youth Conference
-   a declaration in favour of birth control by J. Vermeesch to the Marxist Week of Reflection, the theme of which was: 'Women in the nation': 'As ideas have

converged over the reasons for fear of pregnancy, let us fight together for the right to motherhood.'

The approach of the Presidential elections was to give the question of contraception the scope of national debate. During his electoral campaign François Mitterand approached the question of birth control (as a Communist jounalist, J Derogy, had assured him that it satisfied a real popular need) and claimed to support the repeal of the 1920 law.

At its 1965 conference the MFPF decided to approach the various Parliamentary groups and explain its attitudes in order to inspire the legislators.

The MFPF demanded:

- an amendment to Articles 3 and 4 of the 1920 law which would allow the use of contraception to be legalised (under medical supervision and with no commercial advertising);

- a change in school syllabi, allowing for sex education suited to the pupils' age;

- a liberalising revision of current texts relating to the rights of the woman and the couple.

The relentlessness of the MFPF activists met the election-seeking motivations of the moment and led the Health Ministry to abandon a wait-and-see policy which was increasingly less justifiable as synthetic contraceptives (the pill) had already been available for two years.

These were, of course, theoretically prescribed to control painful and irregular periods but their contraceptive action was no longer a secret to anyone. Nonetheless, it needed a question in the National Assembly for the Health Minister to announce the setting up of a committee to study the consequences of women taking oral contraceptives.

The creation of this committee was the first milestone along the road the authorities would have to travel before recognising contraception. This government committee comprised thirteen professors of medicine and one representative of the Humanities, P H Chombart de Lauwe. This sociologist of world-wide renown, Director of the

Social Ethnology Laboratory at the CNRS (National Scientific Research Centre) had been working with his wife on the problems of the family and the couple for some years. He challenged the fact that a committee of this kind should be totally male and criticised the narrowness of the research brief initially restricted to the medical sphere. Refusing to support the committee's work he withdrew and expressed his point of view in an article in Le Monde on 13 April 1966: 'In contraception it is the very image of the couple, marriage, the family, the roles of the man and the woman which are questioned, and through them, the freedom to choose to have their children; it is a matter of changing the relationships between the sexes and allowing that genuine equality which everybody talks about but few men really want'.

The militants could only rejoice at this distinguished attitude which supported the view the MFPF had been holding for ten years.

But even though public opinion seemed to be increasingly won over to contraception, the people's elected representatives were still 'waiting and seeing'. The few women in the National Assembly who had the additional responsibility of representing their sex proved, through their attitude towards these questions, their lack of independence and the weight of Catholicism even within a secular, Republican structure. In fact when the magazine Elle interviewed eight women deputies only three said they were definitely in favour of the repeal of the 1920 law (two Communists and the one Radical Socialist). The five others were awaiting the verdict of the Synod and contined to defend the 'natural maternal vocation of the woman'.

Turning the debate on contraception into a political debate was not to everyone's taste.

The Confederation Nationale des Associations Familiales Catholiques (National Federation of Catholic Family Associations) expressed its indignation to the press: 'In approaching the subject of birth control, the candidates for the presidency of the Republic are abusing . . . in the hope of winning women's votes, a serious problem which depends only on the conscience of a husband and wife'. For these associations: 'the abolition of the 1920 law . . . would only accentuate the climate of eroticism into which we have fallen and which is so harmful to the young and to domestic stability, doing nothing to reduce abortions'. In the same camp we found Father

Lestapis and Dr Chauchard, stubborn adversaries of Marie-Andrée Weill Halle from the beginning. In publishing Sexual Dignity and the Madness of Contraception Chauchard was hoping to find supporters with whom to share his ideas about the 'blocked-up or pill-bound' woman who could only know the 'sterile love of drug addicts'.

As the legal defender of traditional morality the National Medical Council repeatedly tried to master a trend which was gaining ground.

The debate between the defenders of traditional morality and supporters of contraception was to continue for many years. The bill legalising contraception was, however, passed in December 1967.

28 December 1967: a bitter victory

For the Family Planning Association, the law of December 1967 was very disappointing; it was a bad law. The sole responsibility for contraception was given to the doctors, a prescription was obligatory, and sales were solely through pharmacies.

In the opinion of the MFPF, 'the introduction of clinical records, medical certificate of contraindications, entry in the chemists' register demonstrate the law-makers' intrinsic distrust and the police-state attitude towards female freedom - you could be forgiven for thinking it was being confused with licence. The arrangements about minors confirm the distrust towards those boys and girls who have the most need for legislative provisions which are favourable to their sexual development and their protection'.

The enacting bills which were to come out in the six months following the promulgation of the law were spread out over several years:

-       between February 1969 and March 1972, three decrees were issued governing the manufacture and prescription of contraceptives;

-       then, finally, in April 1972, two decrees were directed at the users: the first, very vague, concerned information centres, the second governed the conditions under which planning centres could operate.

Since December 1967 therefore, contraception was part of the law. In March 1968 the word was introduced into the Academy dictionary, and became part of the language, but the politicians and the doctors were still preventing it from being part of the reality.

For a certain number of MFPF militants the law solved all the problems: others who regarded these measures as inadequate felt that MFPF must not become a social service organisation, but must be an active movement to combat oppression, social inequalities, and exploitation.

Abortion

After 1968 the actions and attitudes of the Movement led activists to become more radical and to take up the struggle for women's rights and free abortion more openly.

Although contraception has been permitted in France since December 1967, a lack of availability and clinic infrastructure meant that it has been accessible only to women who are better-off, better informed, and who have found a competent, open-minded doctor. For this reason abortion often remained the only option in the case of an unwanted pregnancy.

The 1920 law was still in force and although it may not have been enforced in all its vigour it still weighed upon women. The better-off could go abroad or find very expensive solutions in France. The vast majority of French women continued to have abortions, with the guilt, distress, suffering, loneliness and the worst material conditions. Guilty before the law, distressed by the search for a solution and the risk of death, alone because very few would risk helping them because of the fear of legal action, yet they still remained determined to have an abortion.

For fear of being given away, found guilty or even, more simply, humiliated and punished (the reception in hospital was often hostile and the curettages, performed with the aim of dissuasion, were often done without anaesthetic), women only turned to doctors as a very last resort and often they only reached hospital to be mutilated or to die there.

In 1966, the Institut National d'Etudes Demographiques (INED) on the basis of a survey of deaths of an obstetric origin, suggested that there were at least 250,000 illicit abortions and 250 deaths a year (one death for every 1000 women having an abortion; in New York the figure was 0.07 in 1000).

In 1970 the Women's Liberation Movement emerged publicly and set up the Mouvement de Libération de l'Avortement (MLA - Freedom of Abortion Movement); the activists in the MLA moved into action without worrying about 'methods'. Their first provocation was to the law, via the publication on 5 April 1971 in the weekly <u>Le Nouvel Observateur</u> of the Manifesto of 343 women claiming to have committed the offence of abortion.

The trial in Bobigny in 1972 of a minor prosecuted for having an abortion after being raped, and the indictment in 1973 of Annie Ferrey-Martin, a gynaecologist in Grenoble, accused of having perfomed abortions openly at her surgery, regularly brought abortion to the attention of the newspapers.

The women in the MFPF were there: some of them signed the Manifesto, others gave evidence at Bobigny, others issued a communiqué in support of Annie Ferrey-Martin.

In February 1973 the Mouvement de Libération de l'Avortement et de la Contraception (MLAC) was set up: it involved all those who wanted to fight for freedom of abortion and contraception: individual men and women, political parties, associations, trades unions, various groups.

Chiefly under pressure from the feminist movements abortion, although still illegal, began to come out into the open. Let us remember that it was in this climate that the authorities brought the contraception law out of the drawer where it had gathered dust for five years, and issued the first decrees which were to make it applicable to some extent.

Throughout this period developments, took place within the MFPF which were decisive for its future. A new direction became discernible, with the conjunction of two concurrent and irreversible forces: the analysis of the oppression of women carried out by the prime movers in MFPF on the basis of their own daily experience combined with the demands of the feminist movements. MFPF, born earlier as a result of the revolt of some women, became a fighting movement.

Attitudes became radical, political trends asserted themselves. In a motion, at its 1973 Conference MFPF declared that the Movement would perform abortions in its centres, a declaration taken up by the newspapers of the day. It was open warfare, publicly declared.

It was a matter of creating a situation of fact to prove that an abortion performed under satisfactory conditions would not affect women's health. Thanks to the aspiration method, abortion became a lesser medical matter, a simple procedure which many doctors admitted having learned from militant women who were not doctors. Teams were set up to perform abortions with women's groups, doctors of the GIS (Health Information Group), the militants of the MLAC, the MFPF; the women and the teams discussed things together; joint trips to England and the Netherlands were arranged. The MFPF militants had decided to respond openly to women's demands, either by performing the abortions themselves, by giving addresses, or by accompanying trips abroad. Illegality became open.

The film Histoire d'A (The Story of A - a story of a woman's abortion experience) was screened. The showings caused demonstrations; the film was seized by the police and then banned. But it continued to be screened.

Associations and the trades unions, which understood the size of the problem and the social inequalities it revealed, having a greater effect on women who were less well-informed and from deprived social backgrounds, joined the MFPF in this struggle. Information sessions were held in firms, regular clinics were set up there. Teachers and social workers came to the MFPF study groups. Various places, such as the MJCs (Youth and Cultural Centres), the Centres de Protection Infantile (Child Protection Centres) overflowed with demands for operations, debates, information on contraception and abortion.

Between 1972 and 1975 the painful introduction of decrees applying the law on contraception could not satisfy the needs which were becoming increasingly apparent. Decrees psychiatrised and medicalised contraception to the utmost. The MFPF continued to say and say again that contraception is not an illness; that it is not by making it more difficult to obtain that women will become used to the idea of using it; that contraception cannot be forced on anyone; that it is a different outlook on life; that, at any rate, a woman who has decided she does not want a child need not have one; that it is a fundamental right that she is recognising; and that the method she will use in order not to become a mother will be the one that is nearest at hand.

It was in this spirit that in 1974 the MFPF decided,

as a policy priority, to open orthogenic centres and increased its promotional activity and its regular centres.

The aims of the MFPF's orthogenic centres was to prove that information on the right to contraception is essential in order to satisfy the needs of the population, to prove that demedicalisation is necessary in order to make women responsible for their contraception. From then on the MFPF decided to move from the sidelines to centre-stage.

Conditional legalisation of abortion for five years: the MFPF view

In 1975 the new Government passed a law, on a trial basis for five years, which governed the conditions of abortion. This restrictive law only allowed abortion under certain circumstances: for example, there would be no refund from Social Security. The procedures to obtain one were intended to be an 'obstacle course'. But however restrictive the law may have been, many regarded it as a victory, and after it was passed all those various forces which had combined to fight for it disbanded.

Since 1971 the MFPF had been saying 'no law can govern the question of abortion'; it had repeated this when it was consulted by the committee preparing the law for the National Assembly.

It was to go on fighting, virtually alone, for five years.

The MFPF and illegality – the battles

The MFPF conducted the battles on two levels:

- to oblige the authorities to apply the law, however inadequate it may be. It decided to stop performing terminations in its centres, but fought to have abortion departments opened in hospitals;
- to show up the inadequacies of the law. Illegal abortions continued 'every woman who wants an abortion, within or outside the law, must find a response to her request'. The MFPF set to work; under-aged girls, foreign girls or women more than 10 weeks pregnant came to the planning service, certain of finding a response to their request.

From that point onwards and with patience, the MFPF

prepared files in support of its statements and worked towards establishing a fait accompli. Doctors performed abortions beyond the legal limit, clinics and even some hospitals accepted under-age girls without parental consent and foreign women without asking them how long they had been in France, the 'week of thought' which the law provided for was not totally observed. This considerably reduced trips abroad.

This did not mean all was well - far from it. The public sector, by responding inadequately to women's needs, whether in respect of their request for an abortion or for contraception, left things open for the private sector with the abuses which can result - financial abuse above all, over and over again. Also, women were still subject to the doctor's decision as to the method of termination.

In 1978 the MFPF organised an international conference on IVG (voluntary termination of pregnancy), the purpose of which was to prove, by combining different methods, that the torpidity in the application of the IVG law was partly due to the retrograde attitude of the French medical profession which refused to use modern methods shown to be harmless abroad.

All the difficulties encountered by women were to be brought to public attention on the occasion of the MFPF National Sittings on 31 March 1979. Evidence from women and militants from all over France flooded in about the inadequacy of the Veil law, and the unsatisfactory application of the law on contraception: no publicity actually available, cost-free operation for minors not implemented, bad faith apparent on the part of the authorities apart from one or two exceptions, administrative sluggishness, obstruction from hospital departmental heads.

Confident of these criticisms, and refusing to continue responding to the demands arising because of the law on a makeshift basis, the militants once again contacted the trades unions associations and women's groups to demand that the real needs of women be taken into account. The time was right. The Veil law was to be discussed again in Parliament in December 1979. Already in June the European elections had been an opportunity for the Right to take up the subject of respect for life in order to demand limitations to the existing law, which was already restrictive anyway. The powers that be cleverly took up the matter, the Health Minister changed, centres closed, fines and trials followed. These various forms of repression were aimed at women.

Charges against a clinic, started when the law was under discussion, and negative publicity showed the Government's obvious wish to restrict those rights already acquired and to suppress the advantages gained after much struggle on important matters.

Demonstrations began again. The most spectacular was to be the women's march of 6 October: more than 50,000 women demonstrated and claimed in the streets that abortion was a right. The definitive law passed in December 1979 was a huge disappointment for women.

Five years of struggle, action, analysis had only ended in the renewal of the law, with more serious penalties, by a divided Parliament where the Left had been caught in a trap; women of all shades of opionion who attended the Parliamentary discussion of the law came out disgusted by the scorn, peevishness and even stupidity they had heard.

The Government, in the person of the Health Minister, undertook to apply 'the law and nothing but the law'; no more arrangements, no more accommodations. But an unresponsive repression intensified. The doctors were the ones who were punished, and through them, women were affected. The English clinics once again received a large number of French women and the MFPF clinics once again began to be strained under the demands of women in genuine distress, often sent by the hospitals, medical social workers, doctors.

The situation seemed a complete stalemate. One hope: the Presidential elections and a change of government.

May 1981: a change of Government - positive government measures.

In the Autumn of 1981 the Government launched a national publicity campaign on the family planning centres through the media and published brochures giving their addresses and opening hours. These were available in public places (Government offices, Town Halls etc.).

This national publicity campaign was all the more important as it preceded a legal text (PMI circular) showing the Government's desire to make known what existed.

At the beginning of 1982 the Ministry of Women's Rights, which replaced the Ministry of the Status of Women, began to distribute a brochure on contraceptive methods free-of-charge, and a guide to the rights of women. It

Case Study: France

financed a series of courses on 'awareness of sexuality matters' intended for social, medical, para-medical and educational workers, organised by the MFPF as part of its information policy.

In 1982 a memorandum from the National Education Ministry dealt with informing pupils about contraception and the training of teachers in this subject. For the MFPF, all these measures indicating a change of attitude were positive.

Problems

On the other hand, in spite of the promises made during the Presidential campaign and in spite of the Prime Minister's announcement in Paris on 8 March 1982 that abortion would soon be refunded by Social Security, this decision was not shared by all members of the Government, which was evasive. In September the Ministry of Social Affairs even went so far as to say that 'it's a matter of ethics'.

In addition, and since the Spring of 1982, the opponents of abortion ('Let them Live') had been mobilising and exerting pressure against this refund.

Faced with this situation, which it considered unthinkable, the MFPF, the Women's Movement and other organisations decided to arrange a demonstration to prove to the public and the Government that the population was still mobilised around this problem and urged the Government to ensure that the undertakings made were fulfilled.

Refund at last

In spite of the announcement of refunding published on 20 October 1982, the demonstration still went ahead: it was a success.

The decree appeared on 31 December 1982 and it was several months before the refunding became effective.

For the MFPF this was a victory for women, but the Movement is continuing to act in order to obtain the decriminalisation of abortion (reform of the Penal Code under way) but like everything else which affects morality, this demand is encountering huge problems. Attitudes do not develop quickly and today, we can still say that there are many things to do.

Case Study: France

FACTS

1   Contraception

Where it is prescribed

     In 1980 the National Institute for Demographic Studies assessed the number of women between 15 and 49 (i.e. potential users of contraception) at 12 million.

     In France contraceptives are prescribed in the public health sector, in the independent associations sector, and in the professional practice of medicine by GPs and gynaecologists.

     In the public sector the planning centres approved by the Health Ministry are located in hospitals, mother and child protection centres, and municipal clinics.

     In the associations sector contraceptives are prescribed through such organisations as Mutuelle des Etudiants (Students' Friendly Society), Mutuelle des Enseignants (Teachers' Friendly Society), MFPF etc.

     In 1983, 777 planning centres were listed by the Health Ministry, but the majority of them are in urban areas and they do not always open at times which are suitable for those who wish to use them.

     The 30 MFPF orthogenic centres give information and prescribe contraceptives. In 1982 these centres were open on Wednesday afternoons for the young student population, 24 were open at times suitable for working people.

     These 30 centres were open for a total of 30,836 hours in 1982; 45,114 people were seen (including 29,782 under 20 years of age), 52,598 medical acts were performed, 33,449 for people under 20 .

MFPF 1982 survey – use of contraceptives

     In 1982, the MFPF organised a survey on 'contraception from the woman's point of view'. This survey covered a representative sample of the French population. But it must be stressed that the women who agreed to answer the questionnaire (3,133) were already aware of and concerned with contraception.

     At the time of the survey 80% of the women used a method of contraception, 14% had stopped using one and 6% had never used one at all.

If we take account of:

- those women who had stopped using a contraceptive because they wanted a child;
- those who did not have or no longer had sexual relations;
- those who did not need contraception.

we reach a percentage of approximately 6% of women who were not using a contraceptive at the time but were risking unwanted pregnancy. In comparison in the INED 1978 survey this figure was 3%.

We should note that there are some fairly important differences according to the women's ages, especially in the case of the over 45s, some of whom no longer need contraception, and the youngest who had not yet had sexual experience.

The methods used by the women at the time of the survey were:

Pill	42.0%
Coil	20.0%
Diaphragm, sheath, spermicide	7.5%
Other methods	7.0%
Sterilisation	3.0%
No method	19.5%
No answer	1.0%

In the INED 1978 survey 28% of the women took the contraceptive pill and 9% had a coil. There is no way of comparing the data on the other methods as the groupings are different. In an IFOP survey in 1979, 33% took the pill.

On the other hand, as the women interviewed were asked about the contraceptive method they had used most recently, we do know that 94% of them had used at least one method of contraception during their lives, mainly the pill; next came the coil, and then the other methods very far behind.

Publicity

The Government's national publicity campaign in the Autumn of 1981 notified the public of the addresses of the information and family planning centres. The family planning survey carried out some months after this campaign obtained the views of women familiar with contraception.

According to our results,

44% of women had seen the advertisements on TV
43% had heard about them
18% had listened to the radio broadcasts
16% had seen the lists of addresses
15% had not heard anything

These data differ appreciably from those published by the Women's Rights Ministry, which covered the entire population.

Cross-referencing enabled us to determine that the young were least aware of this campaign. Fewer of the young had heard about it, or seen the TV advertisements, perhaps because at their age one watches television less, or at least at that time of day when the advertisements were broadcast. The campaign has most successfully reached the salaried and managerial class group, which included a lot of teachers. It was they who had spotted the lists of addresses of planning centres available in various public places (Post Offices, Town Halls etc) in the largest numbers. The TV and radio broadcasts had basically reached women at home and the oldest women.

Finally, of women's opinion on the suitability or quality of this information campaign: - 93% of women who had seen and heard the campaign thought it useful; 53% thought it useful but inadequate; 29% thought it was good, useful; 11% thought it useful but badly done; 0.5% thought it was not useful, had no point; 0% thought it was shocking, uncalled-for; 5.5% had no opinion; 1% did not answer.

But if it was the women at home and working class women who mainly replied 'good, useful', it was the salaried and managerial women and students who were more likely to say 'useful but inadequate'; they were in favour of the campaign but critical of it.

Alongside this campaign the Ministry for Women's Rights published a brochure on 'Contraception, a Fundamental Right'.

The MFPF survey also gave an indication of the way in which women found out about methods of contraception. An extract from the survey follows.

Case Study: France

Source of contraceptive information according to age.

	Up to 20 years of age	20-29 years of age	30 and over
Friends	51%	38%	28%
School	42%	22%	1%
Parents	33%	20%	4%
Media	19%	23%	23%
Doctor	19%	35%	45%
Planning centres	14%	7%	9%

When the information was obtained

	at the MFPF	outside the MFPF	
First sexual experience:	39%	33%	34%
Adolescence:	18%	13%	15%
When starting a relationship:	7%	11%	10%
After having been afraid of getting pregnant or after a termination:	16%	14%	15%
No personal action:	5%	7%	6%

This survey was the basis of the international conference on 'Contraception from the woman's point of view' organised by the MFPF in December 1982. A publicity brochure on contraceptive methods has been distributed since 1978 at a very low price (5 francs).

Also, the Youth and Sports Ministry, in conjunction with the Ministry for Women's Rights, the Health Ministry and various associations including the MFPF prepared a leaflet aimed at the young, 'J'aime, je m'informe' (I'm in love, I'm finding out), which was distributed free in the Youth Information Centres.

2   Abortion

(See national profile for France)

The restrictions of the 1979 law cause a certain

number of women to be in an illegal position (too late,
minors without parental consent, foreign women). The MFPF
has carried out a survey and an analysis based on 1900
cases in 1982-83 which were sent to the relevant
Ministries, the President of the Republic etc., thus
pursuing its aims in favour of the decriminalisation of
abortion and the withdrawal of the restrictions.

3   Sterilisation

(See national profile for France)

4   Adoption

(see national profile for France)

Catholics are still acting against abortion and in
January 1984 they set up an association 'Magnificat' to
encourage women to continue their pregnancies to full term
and give up the child at birth. In fact French law allows
women to give birth anonymously, which enables them to
renounce their rights to the child which is then handed
over to the Aide Sociale à l'Enfance (Social Aid for
Children - an official body) or to private associations for
adoption, but the number of 'adoptable' children is
decreasing considerably.

5   Infertility

The arrival of new bio-technologies (in-vitro
fertilisation, artificial insemination, surrogate
motherhood etc.) poses serious legal and moral questions.
In fact the technical limitations bring increasingly fewer
arguments against the current limits of ethics.
But infertile women and couples who want a child very
much see these techniques as offering a solution to their
problem and apply pressure to be able to take advantage of
them. But at what price? Associations, whose purpose is
not necessarily altruistic, have already been set up to
satisfy this demand.
The MFPF is currently considering this and some
queries arise, such as:
So far, the principle of organ donation has been
donation without reward (blood, sperm, etc.). Is there not
a danger of this principle being called into question?

Might there not be the risk of financial trading if this became commercial? Might not the rental of a womb lead disadvantaged women to take up this form of 'new trade' to the advantage of well-off women (a new form of prostitution). All the standards associated with the reproduction of the species (couple, family, value of the maternal function, transfer of inheritance, children being brought up by their natural parents, Christian morality, importance of the relationship between the mother and the foetus) are called into question by these techniques. Should we worry about it or should we be pleased?

These questions do not only concern the various ethical committees set up, but all women.

Conclusion

As far as information is concerned, the situation has not improved a great deal in spite of efforts made by the Government when it came to power. Many women do not know their rights and/or do not know where to turn to exercise them. The accent is increasingly placed on conjugal advice rather than on publicity. Furthermore, the Government's family policy, which tends very much to encourage motherhood, seems to acknowledge women's rights to freedom of choice but is based on the demographic situation (which is regarded as worrying) and patriotic responsibility.

Even though contraception may seem to be recognised as a basic right, many women from underprivileged backgrounds or rural areas cannot exercise this right. On the other hand, the right to freedom of choice to have a child or not does not stop at contraception.

As long as Article 317 of the Penal Code exists, as long as voluntary sterilisation is not accepted, as long as contraceptive publicity and methods are not widely available to all women and men, this will only be a limited right. Can we then call it a basic right?

Recognition of the fundamental right

Although there is no official French text which explicitly recognises that the right to decide whether or not to have children is a fundamental right, in signing the resolutions of the Council of Europe, France has not wanted to refuse to acknowledge the existence of this right. Nonetheless, abortion is still part of the penal code, which makes it a criminal offence unless it is practised under the terms of the law of December 1979; only the repeal of this clause of the penal code will be a genuine and complete recognition of this right.

On the other hand, for the majority of European countries voluntary sterilisation is a method of family planning. By construing 'planning' methods only to include reversible methods of contraception, France can sign declarations with a clear conscience while still failing to offer men and women the number of options available in other countries. Thus there is some ambiguity here concerning the meaning of the terms used, exploited for political reasons.

Since 1968 many texts have been passed moving towards a recognition of this right: these have been dealt with in another part of this document. The amendments which follow provide an alternative means by which this right may be exercised and tries to explain their limitations and propose solutions by which to cope with them.

Access to Contraception is a principle guaranteed by the law. There is reimbursement by social security, free for women who are minors and who have no national insurance, in the planning centres. However, there is one group which is overlooked, the 18-20 year olds who are legally of age but have no national insurance in their own right if they do not work and thus depend on their parents. In most planning centres until quite recently, the 18-20 year olds were included with minors but budgetary restraint has led to a tightening-up and many cases of refusal.

In principle women ought to be able to choose between private medicine and the public centres. In effect in 1983 there were 777 centres for 12 million women between 15 and 49 years old, ie. approximately 1 centre for every 15,000 women. Because of the widespread financial restrictions it is unlikely that any new centres are planned. Moreover, decentralisation (recently enacted) has put the centres in the charge of the county councils (departmental) which are controlled on the whole by right-wing majorities. Thus there is the tendency to stop 'unprofitable' opening times, which works to the advantage of private medicine. This reduction in the length of opening hours makes the position of the freelance staff (particularly doctors) increasingly precarious and less attractive financially. Everything thus pushes these doctors towards the private sector or established public-sector posts. Also, even though the work is interesting, they never stay long in the centres, and this constant turnover is unsatisfactory both for the women and the centre teams.

We have pointed out that centres in mountainous, rural areas or where the inhabitants are very scattered are non-existent, and these are the areas with a chronic lack of general practitioners and gynaecologists in particular. The structure the law provides for is far too heavy in terms of finance and staff to be practicable everywhere, and other forms of funding the system ought to be considered.

The problem of opening times is based on two opposing requirements: those of the clientele and those of the centre staff. If the centre staff have not really accepted that the right to contraception is not only restricted to existing mothers, but that the young and sometimes even the very young may have a sex life and want contraception, that working women may wish to come in after work or during their break times, very little effort will be made. And at present many centres are still not open when young people are free. It is true that school hours vary a great deal and the traditional Wednesday afternoon off is gradually disappearing in favour of Saturday, and in our MFPF centres we have had to alternate different opening times in order to try to cater for the demand. What is more serious, however, is the fact that there are still many towns, small or medium in size but having secondary education facilities (for 14-18 year-olds), which have no planning centre.

It is not our business here to take the public side in the debate between public and private medicine. At the MFPF we primarily want women to choose the solution which suits them best. But we want them to have a quality medical service. At the moment doctors' training consists of only four hours (not compulsory) on contraception, and in subsequent training contraception is rarely brought up. Doctors are thus subject to pressure from the pharmaceutical companies' representatives (which has led to a vast prescription of mini-pills) when they do not seek additional training on their own initiative. In our view this represents a very serious gap which often culminates in applications for abortion or a difficult sex life.

Our proposals are as follows:

- Bring the 18-20 year olds with no personal national insurance out of the cold and find a legal solution for them, as they are covered by the contributions paid by their parents.

- Take more systematic account of contraception in the various budgets, in view of the fact that this contraception is at various levels, particularly through the setting-up of lighter structures, mini-centres or mobile vehicles.

- Give priority of access to the public centres to the young because contraception can only be free in these centres. This really means synchronising the timetables of educational establishments and the centres or mini-centres. Propose a type of reception which meets the youngsters' requirements (we come back to this in the section on information). We did not want to choose between specific structures for young people or integrated structures; for us this is not the nub of the problem. It is more a question of the spirit in which the centres operate, the quality of the reception, the locations and the times of opening.

- Provide both <u>theoretical</u> and <u>practical</u> training for medical and paramedical personnel and further training not only in contraceptive techniques but also sexuality as a whole. None of this can be achieved without the political will. If this tends towards a greater respect for women's choice, we hope it will make itself heard more.

That commercial advertising of contraceptives be banned by law does not seem contestable to us. But the fact that so little has been done to implement the broad principles expressed in 1973 - 'information on contraception . . . is a <u>national responsibility</u>', - and in 1979: 'information on the problems of life is a <u>national obligation</u>' - appears very serious to us. No or very little money has been made available; no access to the media was forthcoming until the initiative of the Women's Rights Ministry in 1981. We welcomed this initiative with hope; for us it had a symbolic value. We knew it responded to a great demand, but a few months later the lists of addresses and the TV advertisements had disappeared; the

television discussions and information broadcasts are
non-existent. We cannot understand why lists of the
centres' addresses have still not appeared in many
departments to this day. And yet in 1980 a Minister
offered to distribute this list to pharmacists, school
health staff and a 1983 circular stated that the opening
times and activities of the centres must be brought to the
notice of the public through bill-posting, putting up
direction signs etc.

Travelling through France the eye is rarely attracted
by a sign pointing to a centre, and as for lists of
addresses, how many of us can actually find one in a public
place today? Looking for the details about the centres in
a telephone directory can sometimes be an instructive
experience when one finds one has to look under health
centre or hospital. As for the term 'planning centre', it
often needs additional explanation.

How can we explain this situation when official texts
exist? Why are these texts not implemented? What
facilities does a Government have to implement the texts it
passes or draws up? It seems difficult to lay all the
blame on budgets. Nothing can be done without money, that
is true, but the cost of some forms of action (posting,
signposting) really is minimal. We have the impression
that information is of no interest to our elected
representatives and officials; whereas the law insists on
information, the majority of the finance goes to
counselling. The training provided for in the texts refers
to 120 hours for information activities and 400 hours plus
two years' practical for counselling. Information thus
seems to be a minor activity. Is this not rather a
devaluation of the importance of information? Our
experience has shown us that information is not just a
matter of pouring out one's knowledge to people; a large
part of the problems women have in controlling their
fertility comes from the fact that the information they
have received is badly put, badly suited to their needs, or
else did not give them the wherewithal to take their own
initiative.

There is therefore no agreement in the country on the
content of this information. The outcry caused,
particularly in the Catholic press, by a leaflet intended
for young people, 'J'aime, Je m'informe' (I'm in love, I'm
finding out), which was distributed officially, illustrates
this very well. For many people, telling the young about

sexuality and contraceptive methods incites them to have sexual relations, or is even considered as incitement to debauchery, and this is what the parents, whatever their religious and political beliefs, find the most difficult to accept.

The MFPF has always wanted to be a body which makes proposals, and since the Left came to power in 1981 we have conveyed many proposals, particularly those concerning information, to the appropriate Ministries.

We are recommending:

- That information genuinely be provided within the existing infrastructures, and in a form which presents the whole subject of contraception in its social context rather than merely its technical aspects.

- That it be given as often as possible in a collective fashion with the active participation of the clients.

- That it be offered through associations other than the MFPF.

- That it be financed by global agreements, not on the basis of hours of upkeep but on a report of activities, or on specific innovative or experimental projects such as information campaigns in rural or disadvantaged areas. (It is not enough to finance the start of a project like that of a minibus which travelled through the department of Maine et Loire, or a survey to find out the most suitable ways of giving information to the people in a rural area such as Montluçon, but to ensure that the findings are then implemented.)

- That information be provided regularly via the media. This information should make contraception accessible to all women without obligation or restriction or making it a moral issue. It should make women aware of their rights and options. It cannot be separated from information about pregnancy, childbirth, the place of the child in society, abortion, or sexuality. It should be directed at everyone. It should also have the aim of raising questions, i.e. allowing criticism, because there is no 'correct' method and the choice of a means of contraception for a woman is hers. Contraception is a way of life and information should allow freedom to use it or not according to an individual's case history and living conditions.

- That such information be provided by all those who have chosen educational jobs. Training relating to sexual rights and contraceptive methods should be given in all medical, paramedical and educational professions. In many cases the MFPF can undertake this training, as has been the case for the last two years with the awareness courses financed by the Women's Rights Ministry.

The availability of family planning literature

We have noted that the relevant Ministries' willingness to make up for the lack of information by publishing brochures is limited. 'J'aime, je m'informe' is now not so well distributed by the authorities, who are likely to give in to the moralising pressure of the Catholic community. Is its distribution going to be increased?

Several books on sexuality have been published, in response to the popularity and because of the profitability of the subject. Nevertheless, we do think there is a lack of small, reasonably priced books which in particular answer the questions young people ask themselves. The MFPF has published and re-issued a brochure on contraception which sells for 5 francs and is very much in demand.

Sterilisation: We have noted the legal void relating to sterilisation as a contraceptive method and the ambiguity of the French position vis-à-vis other European countries. Our Association does not have any legal proposals to make. We would like sterilisation to be available to men and women within the social security reimbursement system, on condition that they are informed of the current virtual irreversibility of the operation. We object to the fact that, at present, what is refused in a hospital is possible in a private clinic; that what is refused some women is forced upon others; that sterilisation is available to those who are able to pay.

Abortion: is currently legal only under very specific conditions which we regard as restrictive. Nonetheless we have pointed out and recognised the efforts made by the present Government to have the law applied positively in hospitals. The existing texts are valid and if always applied in the spirit in which they were drafted the position of women requiring an abortion would be more satisfactory.

Currently, women are still not able to choose the place in which they have an abortion. They must have it where the first appointment is offered within a reasonable period of time, whatever the distance from their home or their financial circumstances. Every day in our MFPF premises we receive women who have not been able to find a bed in a hospital or who have been obliged to go to a private clinic. For some, of course, the choice of the private sector is a real choice, but not for all. The obstacles are often financial, the clinics do not always operate the 'one third' payment system (the women have to pay the full price for the operation and claim the money back afterwards); costs are often excessive and the possibility of medical assistance paying for the abortion not always guaranteed. The conditions under which medical assistance is allocated have become very strict, and women are rarely reimbursed the 20% of the cost to which they are entitled; and anonymity for young women (18-20) is not always guaranteed. However, there are no problems for women <u>without</u> national insurance (who are few in number).

There are restrictions in addition to legal ones. The ten weeks of pregnancy specified by law are often reduced to eight weeks on various pretexts and the presence of one parent is sometimes required in addition to parental approval in the case of minors.

We are thus asking that:

- all the texts governing voluntary termination of pregnancy be applied in reality;
- action be taken to check that they are;
- the hospitals' intake capacity be adequate even during staff holidays;
- the practice of early abortions be extended and that they be performed in comfortable and attractive places such as family planning centres.

We want doctors to be trained in abortion techniques and in every abortion clinic for their to be some doctors, at least, who perform terminations right up to the legal limit.

On the other hand, we denounce the inadequacy of this law which forces thousands of women a year to seek abortions in those countries of Europe where the law is less restrictive. We have passed to the relevant ministries two studies each concerned with approximately 2000 illegal abortions. Some of these applications could have been legal if women and doctors were better informed, but there will always be applications which cannot be dealt with within the legal limits. Studies carried out in other countries in Europe confirm that whatever the state of information services, which undoubtedly encourage early applications, there are always late applications as a result of changes in circumstances (e.g. desertion by the partner) or problems of attitudes (e.g. fear of parents). But whatever the improvements, they will not solve the basic problem which is and remains the criminalisation of abortion. Only the repeal of Article 317 of the Penal Code and regulations on the performance of voluntary terminations will allow the right of free choice truly to be recognised.

The struggle against infertility

The services enabling men and women to make decisions on the number of children they have includes infertility treatment.

It is said that a significant proportion of cases of so-called secondary infertility are the result of untreated infections. It is therefore absolutely essential for people to be informed about the risks of complications if even mild infections go untreated and to institute proper preventive measures. We are sure that it is often at the time of an application for contraception that these infections are discovered, and, apart from serious cases, it should be possible to treat and deal with them in all the planning centres (which is not the case at present). The development of new techniques means that certain forms of infertility can be treated by means of artificial insemination: in-vitro and in-vivo fertilisation. There is no legislation on this subject as yet. At present, medical staff alone have the power to choose who is eligible for such treatment. These techniques do, however, pose serious legal and ethical questions. In 1983 the President of the Republic appointed an 'Ethics Committee for the Sciences of

Life and Health' composed of 36 'sensible people' (only 8 women).

For the MFPF it is apposite to think about the use to which these technologies may be put. At present a woman's body is still required in order successfully to make a child, and the freedom of decision when faced with a particular technique rests with the woman. We should not, however, under-estimate the power of social pressure which does not really recognise a woman other than as a mother.

But the possibility of creating an individual 'outside' the womb is no longer science fiction. Even though this may be a complete liberation of the female condition, it also means the possibility of all kinds of operations to modify genetic data. There is then the risk of eugenic practices designed to suit the political or economic objectives of Governments. There is also a risk for the child - the result of an overwhelming desire on the part of parents who will have invested so much that the price paid to achieve it will not bear failure or disappointment.

At the end of all these techniques, what will become of this product, which is a child?

The existence of an Ethics Committee is important. However, it is essential for the feminist movements to be represented on it, to ask specific questions and exert some control. For these movements are at present the only guarantee that genuine attention is paid to the rights of individuals. They have always fought to impose limits on the right of the state to intervene in fertility control, as is shown in their historic struggle for contraceptive and abortion rights.

The MFPF will take care to see that the rights which women have won with difficulty and struggle will not, in their name, be diverted from the objective they are pursuing.

CONCLUSION

Regarding information, the position has not greatly improved despite Government efforts. Many women still do not know their rights and/or do not know where to go to exercise them. In addition, the emphasis is placed on marriage counselling rather than information. Furthermore, the Government's family policy, which strongly encourages procreation, seems to recognise the right of women to free choice but leans towards patriotic responsibility and the demographic situation which is considered disturbing.

As long as Article 317 of the Penal Code exists, as long as voluntary sterilisation is not accepted, as long as information and means of contraception are not widely available to men and women, the right will be a limited one. Can we then call it a fundamental right?

History and Politics of Planned Parenthood Laws in Poland
M Kozakiewicz

The idea of planned parenthood in Poland has a long history. In 1930, a group of progressive physicians and writers (Boy-Zelenski, Boguszewska, and Krzywicka) started a campaign to abolish the prohibition on induced abortion, and began a movement dedicated to disseminating information on how to prevent unwanted pregnancy. In the event, the campaign failed, though out of this activity was born the 'League for the Reform of Morals', which soon changed its name to 'The Society for Conscious Motherhood and the Reform of Morals'. In 1934, the congress of this society proposed a resolution to the Polish government concerning sex reform, birth control, and the legalisation of induced abortion on economic/social grounds, to be performed in hospitals.

From the beginning this society was continually attacked by the Roman Catholic Church, though gaining many adherents from among the intelligensia. After 1935, following the death of Marshal Pilsudski, Polish politics became increasingly right-wing, showing a tendency towards fascism. The significance and power of the Church increased accordingly, to the detriment of the Society for Conscious Motherhood, which suffered from lack of funds. The attacks of churchmen and reactionary politicians ceased with the outbreak of World War II.

In brief, between the years 1932-39, the idea of family planning in Poland was always linked with progressive, liberal-democratic and left-wing political circles, attacked by the right and the Church, and ignored by or producing hostility among the poorly-educated working class - to which its message was principally addressed.

Following World War II, the situation changed radically. Firstly, Poland suffered an enormous loss of population (6 million: 644,000 in combat; 5.4 million due to occupation terror and extermination). In addition, changes in the Polish frontiers and immigration/emigration produced a decline in the resident population from 35 million in 1939, to 21 million in 1945. A consequence of these events was a consciousness of the need for a greater population and a high spontaneous birthrate.

After the war, Poland's population was 21 million; by 1950, 25 million; and by 1960, 30 million; reaching the pre-war level of 36 million by 1984. Although psychologically desirable to Poles this increase imposed enormous economic strains on the Polish economy, particularly after 1955. The State had been unable to secure suitable housing, education, or health for a growing population living with war devastation. The race between economic growth and increasing population has been to the detriment of the latter, leading to the first signs of consciousness in government circles, traditionally antagonistic to planned parenthood, of the need for a slower population growth-rate.

The founding of the Communist state in Poland diminished the traditionly unlimited power of the Roman Catholic Church, partly through the constitutional separation of Church and State, and through removing from Church influence certain educational and health services. As a result, the legalisation of contraception and abortion was made possible, and the family planning movement began to establish the first services - something which would have been impossible before the war. By 1957, family planning was well established in Poland.

As with other Communist societies, Poland placed great stress on mass education, and illiteracy was rapidly eradicated in the 5 years following the end of the war. The level of educational attainment, as measured by number of years of schooling per capita, doubled in the towns and quadrupled in the villages. By the 1960s, urban youth received 12 years of schooling, village youth 10 years. This development exposed the masses to information on sexual matters, including contraception, which has stimulated cultural changes among today's adult generation. Four other legal reforms which preceded this (legalisation of divorce; lowering of the age of majority from 21 to 18 years; introduction of secular marriage as the only legal form; introduction of legal equality of children born in and out of wedlock) have together changed the character of Polish society.

In recognition of these changes which had occurred since 1945, the Seym (government) of the Polish People's Republic passed a law, in 1956, legalising abortion on social as well as medical grounds. One year later, due to the initiative of a group of physicians (Bednardski, Kasprzak, Bulska, Beaupre, Brzozowska), social workers (Musialowa, Parzynska), and the pre-war activist, Krzywicka, the Society for Conscious Motherhood was re-established in November 1957. From the beginning the role of this Society was to act as a 'lightning conductor' drawing attacks away from the Government. Predictably, the passing of the abortion law had provoked hostile counter-propaganda from the Church, albeit within the Church's walls - during sermons. At this time, the existence of a non-governmental organisation to inform people of their legal rights to abortion, to organise sex education, to found the first family planning clinics, to educate gynaecologists and physicians, to develop the production of contraceptives, was tactically convenient for a liberal and sympathetic government. For it could re-direct attacks from the Church to this organisation.

Initially, the Society for Conscious Motherhood was dominated by the medical profession (principally gynaecologists) focussing its attention on abortion and contraception. By the early 1960s, the Society widened its scope to include family health and well-being and sex education as basis for marriage and family life - issues which eventually overshadowed abortion and contraception in its work. New individuals joined this society at this time (sexologists: Imielinski, Jaczewski, Godlewski; sociologists and educationalists: Markowska, Kozakiewicz and Majda; paediatricians: Gornicki and many others).

However, this broader front made the situation more difficult for the Society. Cohabitation, sexuality and even reproduction were matters which still caused considerable embarrassment not only to the Church but to the majority of the population of all educational levels. Puritanism was also a feature of Polish communism, advocates of which were remarkably similar to the Church in their stance on sexual matters, while being diametrically opposed to it on all others.

During the 1960s and 1970s, State censorship increasingly concerned itself with 'immoral' and 'obscene' publications, including the publications of the Society (which had in 1970 changed its name to the Family Planning Association). This was to become a greater obstacle to the work of the Association than the attacks of the Church. It would take many years to eradicate old-fashioned prejudices and taboos relating to such issues as premarital intercourse, masturbation, homosexuality and contraception for adolescents, not only among the general population but among the ruling authorities.

Partly as a result of the new legislation, and due to other demographic changes at the end of the 1960s, population growth had dropped to 0.7-0.8%; and the live birth rate had declined from 30 per thousand population in 1956 to 18.7 in 1968. This provoked some concern both on the part of the Government and the Church. In 1970, the Government of Edward Gierek had come to power, with some covert assistance from the Church. Part of its programme for the accelerated economic development of Poland included a pronatalist population policy. This policy was proclaimed in the mass media in the form of an arithmetic formula for the model family: 2+3. Women bearing 8 and 12 children were designated 'mother heroes' in the media and by the Church. The combination of a pronatalistic policy based on incentives, an upturn in the Polish economy, and a period of high numbers in the population in the most fertile age range, produced a surge in the population growth rate of over 1% per annum between 1971 and 1983.

Increasing economic problems since 1975 have brought the State yet closer to the Church for political reasons. Under pressure from Gierek personally, the Polish FPA was forced to change its name to 'Family Development Association' (Towarzystwa Rozwoju Rodziny (TRR)). In 1976, the paper supply to TRR for publications was cut (36 tons per annum). Due to a local government ban, it became more difficult to collect and receive donations from individuals and organisations on which the TRR depended. The import of contraception was curtailed and national production discouraged, in spite of the protestations of the TRR.

During 1976-77 contraceptives became virtually unavailable, with the exception of a small supply from the TRR-owned factory 'Securitas', which was having problems obtaining raw materials. The State pharmaceutical distribution centre (Cefarm) refused to distribute spermicides and the IUDs manufactured by Securitas under the pretext of lack of demand. Such pressures created grave financial difficulties for TRR, limiting in turn the availability of sex education and family planning services throughout the country (see Appendix 3). A course entitled 'Preparation for Family Life', introduced in 1974 as an optional subject for more than 2000 schools, was the result of intensive work by TRR professionals. However, the contents were increasingly challenged and cut down through the pressure of the Church, which argued that its contents were contrary to Catholic conscience and teaching.

The financial base of TRR has also been undermined during the 1980s through administrative reforms ordered by the Government, which multiplied the number of counties in Poland from 17 to 49. This placed a legal obligation on all national organisations to create a branch for each county, increasing the costs of administration 2.5 times. The reform was in fact aimed at weakening the power of local government in favour of greater central control.

With the impending economic crisis in Poland, accompanied by social and political tensions which began to take the form of underground opposition to the regime, the Government looked to the Church for yet further support (or at least its neutrality). The area of maternal and family health was chosen as a suitable platform for State-Church cooperation. During 1978-9, there even emerged politicians of secular persuasion who supported the de-legalisation of abortion, discussing alternative drafts within the mass media. TRR took action to defend the existing legislation and to raise support for it from among the enlightened public.

In August 1980, the famous socio-political earthquake hit Poland in the form of the Gdansk strikes and the formation of the movement 'Solidarity' shortly afterwards. The umbrella of Solidarity was quickly used as a means for previously underground highly reactionary Roman Catholic organisations to campaign openly. For example, 'Gaudium Vitae' and 'Care for Life' began a merciless campaign against all contraception in general, and TRR in particular. Solidarity, itself, with the exception of some branches in southern Poland, did not take a position on demographic and medical issues connected with family planning and sex education. Unfortunately however, the close relationship it had with the Church permitted free space for anti-family planning activities by certain of its members. One result of this activity was the total ban on the Preparation for Family Life school course in 1981 by the Ministry of Education. This conservative offensive was directed at all three fields of TRR activity: contraception, abortion and secular sex education, with the assistance of anti-abortion publications imported from the

United States. The mass media appeared to be at the disposal of the anti-family planning movement at this time, and members of TRR were vilified and physically threatened. Due to this onslaught, the TRR was slandered as a member of a 'baby-killing mafia based in London' and one-third of its members left the organisation. By 1981-2, TRR had reached the threshhold of bankruptcy.

Through the efforts of several members of TRR to utilise the media in a counter-propaganda exercise, the situation was turned around. During its heaviest battle, TRR published its 'Statement on Family Planning in Poland' (Appendix 2) and began to make use of the news and television media to challenge the stance of the Church.

Following the introduction of martial law in December 1981 (lifted July 1983), many organisations including Gaudium Vitae and Care for Life, were proscribed. This brought attacks on TRR to an abrupt end. Ironically, the years 1982-3 saw a record number of births (see Appendix 1) which came to be recognised by the Government as a further threat to efforts to restore economic stability. As a result, the Government slowly and discreetly adopted an antinatalist population stance. TRR began to receive grants from the Ministry of Health which soon made up 50-60% of its budget. This permitted the establishment of new clinics and counselling centres. Resumption of paper supplies, partly from donations from other FPAs and the IPPF, permitted the re-publication of educational materials.

The TRR remains the major provider of family planning and sex education services in Poland in spite of attempts to found counter-organisations in the same field under the auspices of the Church.

Conclusions and TRR recommendations for the enhancement of family planning in Poland

The de jure situation regarding family planning is believed to be satisfactory, though vigilance is necessary to ensure that no restrictive revisions proposed by anti-family planning groups are considered.

However, the TRR recommends that the Seym (or Ministry of Health) draft new laws to cover voluntary sterilisation, AID, and the rights of adolescents to contraceptive services without the permission of parents.

The de facto situation is characterised by serious

deficiencies in the availability of contraceptives and related information materials. Therefore, the Government might consider developing the national production of contraceptives (oral contraceptives, IUDs and condoms), and making up the shortfall in volume and variety by greater import from other countries (condoms from the DDR, Czechoslovakia; orals from Hungary, Yugoslavia or South Korea) as is feasible under the present economic circumstances.

The present low demand for contraception due to the ideological pressure of the Church on the population could be countered by better public information concerning citizens' rights in this area.

The production of condom vending machines for installation in public places is believed to constitute one solution to the problem of poor access to supplies.

The development of a wider network of counselling centres and clinics could be achieved by obliging all existing State-provided 'Mother Care centres' to also offer contraceptives and counselling.

Regarding sex education, the de jure situation is also satisfactory. However, it is necessary to ensure that reactionary school teachers do not restrict the teaching of the full sex education curriculum in secondary schools. It is also necessary to publish better educational materials both for teachers to use with their pupils and to educate teachers themselves.

A system of professional preparation for teachers in this area must be developed.

Conclusion

The pluralistic character of Polish society must be taken into account when dealing with this subject, for example, when preparing educational materials. Sexuality, sex education and family planning must be subjects of public consensus rather than confrontation, subject to open debate, where individual convictions and differences in attitudes can be taken into account.

Case Study: Poland

APPENDIX 1:   Demographic Statistics for 1975-1982

Pop Total	Marriages	Divorces	Live Births	Death Rate	Pop Growth Rate	Infant Mortality per 1000 live births
'000			per 1000 population			
34022	9.7	1.2	18.9	8.7	10.2	25.1
34362	9.5	1.1	19.5	8.8	10.7	24.0
34698	9.4	1.2	19.1	9.0	10.1	24.5
35010	9.3	1.0	19.0	9.3	9.7	22.5
35257	9.0	1.1	19.5	9.2	10.3	21.3
35578	8.6	1.1	19.5	9.9	9.6	21.3
35902	9.0	1.1	18.9	9.2	9.7	20.5
36227	8.7	1.3	19.4	9.2	10.2	20.4

M Kozakiewicz (1984)

APPENDIX 2:

Extracts from Statement made by the Praesidium of the Polish Family Development Association 1980

Family planning in Poland

The publication of a revised edition of the TRR statement: 'On Family Planning, Contraception and Abortion in Poland' has been inspired by several recent developments:

The ending of the 5 year plan 1976-1980 and the preparation of the next 5 year plan 1981-1985, in which the demographic situation is used in general planning and planning of social policy.

The present situation in Poland has a negative influence on the family situation and the level of services provided, among them the public health services. The main objective of our Association is to improve the service.

The pressure from different conservative centres is constantly increasing. They aim to use the period of present difficulties to extort from the authorities different concessions and the revision of existing progressive legislation in the realm of family planning by making the access to contraception more difficult - especially for young people - and by restricting or even abolishing the existing laws on abortion and divorce.

The demographic situation of the country

The last two 5-year plans brought for Poland a very positive demographic balance, which was achieved without restriction of abortion and contraception laws, maintaining full human rights in the domain of family planning.

The real danger for demographic development and existing positive trends in the birthrate lies not in continuation of the same legal conditions for abortions and contraception, but in worsening the economic and social situations of families. If this tendency continues and dramatically worsens, one can foresee a gradually declining birthrate in Poland. But this will happen in spite of contraception and legalised abortion.

Case Study: Poland

The situation in the field of contraception and abortion

It is not in Poland's interest to increase the number of unwanted and accidentally conceived children born under constraint and necessity. It is instead interested in the growth of the numbers of wanted children brought into the world by their parents.

Abortion should be carried out only as an emergency method of fertility regulation; only when contraception has failed; and when serious health and socio-economic factors affect the woman in the case of an unwanted child. The legalisation of abortion - recently introduced in many non-socialist countries, including Austria, Denmark, France, FRG, Finland, Norway, Sweden and UK - is not equivalent to recognition of abortion as a routine method of birth control, but is a recognition of the right of each woman to freely make decisions about her own body and fertility. The number of abortions in Poland is decreasing.

The only efficient way of reducing the number of abortions further is wider availability of information and accessibility of contraception. Countries with restrictive abortion laws now have an increase in the number of illegal abortions, of peri-abortion mortality, and an increase in the number of children dependent on the State.

Therefore, the Praesidium of TRR must stress emphatically that the situation regarding contraception in our country is alarming. In the second half of 1973 and at the beginning of 1976 there was total non-availability of contraceptives in Poland. Nationwide investigations carried out by TRR in 1978 showed a periodical and continuous shortage in quantity and quality of different kinds of contraceptives.

We have in Poland only two brands of oral pills. There is a possibility of importing oral pills from Hungary, (where there are 8 brands) produced in cooperation with Gedeon Richter Ltd.

The IPPF in London tested the quality of Polish condoms and found that 60-80% from the sample were deficient - leaking - while by international standards not more than 10% of condoms should be deficient. The TRR is proposing the import of condoms from Czechoslovakia, which produces condoms conforming to international standards of quality.

In spite of economic difficulties and necessary limitations on importation, the contraceptives which cannot be produced nationally should be imported from abroad, applying the same principle by which important drugs for the protection of citizens' health and well-being are imported.

APPENDIX 3

Statement by the Polish Society for Family Planning Central Body on Contraception in Poland (1977)

A policy on contraception is one of the elements of the state's social policy and an expression of its support for:

- women's rights and the elimination of one of the last relics of the epoch of women's oppression;

- comprehensively-conceived family health and welfare as the fundamental cell of the socialist society;

- the happy childhood and youth of new generations through planning and the potentially most beneficial conditions for their life and development;

- a demographic development of the country conforming to the public interest and within the planned needs of the socio-economic development.

Although legislation on abortion and contraception in Poland is progressive, the birthrate has been increasing since 1970 and is now one of the highest in Europe: 1970, 8.5 per thousand, 1971, 9.4, 1972, 9.6, 1974, 10.2. Similarly, the number of live births increased in the same period from 16.6 to 18.4. (The Central Statistical Board 1975.)

The increase in births, noted since 1970, has proved the correctness of the policy carried out by the State. It consists of increasing motivation to have children through better family and maternal care, and by means of securing improved living conditions for the population as a whole.

In 1972, the number of children per woman of fertile age in Poland was 2.07 in urban and 2.97 in rural areas.

The Polish Society for Family Planning Central Board must clearly emphasise that the constant deficit and recently the almost complete lack of contraceptives during 1975-1976 (condoms, hormonal preparations, diaphragms, etc,) caused serious social harm and must have affected the health of Polish women by making abortion the only widely acceptable method of birth control.

According to the above mentioned CSB studies of 1972, 61.3% of women in the fertile age group in urban areas use a method of contraception and only 50.3% in rural areas. It is no wonder therefore that every third woman in towns and every tenth woman in rural areas resorted to abortion.

It is especially important to provide a knowledge of contraception and contraceptive methods for young people, both male and female. It is becoming more common for young people to start a pre-marital sex-life early and therefore they are apt to resent the consequences of their own complete ignorance of contraception.

Physicians agree that abortions are more harmful to nulliparous women than to multiparous women, frequently giving rise to infertility.

The conviction that knowledge of contraception would encourage pre-marital sexual relations among the masses is unjustified. Such relations already exist - the knowledge of contraception will certainly diminish the threat of accidental pregnancy.

There is no reason for recognising any contraceptive method as the 'leading' one or as requiring preference in recommendations by the health service organisers. The health service should see that women are informed in detail about the degree of reliability of all contraceptive methods and that the chosen method is accessible. Also, to provide honest information about the drawbacks of individual contraceptives - without alarming exaggeration - is one of the necessary premises of educational/information activities in that respect. The final decision on the choice of a contraceptive method belongs to the couple themselves. The point is to make the couple able to take a conscious decision, based upon sound knowledge in this sphere of life, supported if possible, by advice from competent medical staff.

The real accessibility of contraception depends on making it obligatory that contraception counselling services be available within all related medical facilities such as women's consulting clinics, medical cooperatives and hospital gynaecological wards, and not only in specialised Central or Provincial Polish Society for Family Planning clinics. Training of all physicians in contraception is necessary. It should begin at the undergraduate medical educational level and be continued in postgraduate education.

The Development of Planned Parenthood in the United Kingdom
P Meredith

There is no written Constitution in the United Kingdom and no other explicit legal codification of the right to determine the number and spacing of children. However, a number of laws created to permit and encourage individuals to take responsibility for contraception by facilitating access to methods in effect display continuing Government commitment to the above principle.

This situation has come about only through a long tradition of pressure-group struggle to encourage successive Governments to recognise their responsibility to ensure that the mental and physical health, particularly of the female population, is maintained.

Amidst controversy, the first private birth control clinics opened in 1921. Another 53 years passed before the British Government took responsibility for the provision of free-of-charge family planning services. Prior to the 1920s, a Victorian attitude ensured that both sexuality and childbirth were taboo subjects, preventing any discussion of birth regulation. The patriarchal Victorian ideology prohibited any consideration of contraception on the grounds that sexual enjoyment divorced from procreation would undermine the family and the contract of marriage. This belief was founded on a conception of the female as fundamentally corrupting and in need of male control. Contraception would therefore facilitate female infidelity, and subvert the familial process of male inheritance of property.

The notion of sexual pleasure per se as destructive or corrupting of morals was reflected in the teachings of the highly influential Christian churches. The law of God confirmed the connection between sexuality and procreation. The medical profession reinforced this attitude in its capacity as guardian both of health and morality. The powerful influence of the Church and medical the profession within Parliament ensured that the 'anti-sex' status quo was legally sanctioned.

Impetus for change stemmed from a combination of changing economic conditions and legislative changes which guaranteed educational rights to children, and protected them from dangerous employment. Widespread unemployment in the late 19th century increased levels of poverty to the extent that the working class became a threat to the status quo.(1)

Children became an economic burden to poor families partly because of protective legislation which forbad their employment before a certain age, and gave access to education. These factors made family limitation a physical necessity. By the turn of the century, progress in perinatal care also led to a reduction in mortality which increased family size. Consequently, methods of family limitation such as coitus interruptus and illegal abortion produced a decline in the birthrate before any organised attempt to provide birth control services.

The first signs of family limitation came from the middle classes who took advantage of an increasing commercial sector which offered pamphlets and other literature on condoms, spermicides, Dutch caps and abortifacients.(2)

By the end of the First World War, due to the increasing incidence of veneral diseases, the most popular method of contraceptive was the use of the condom. The use of the condom was further encouraged by technological advances in rubber production shortly after 1918.

Other impetus for a birth control movement came from middle-class pressure groups concerned with poverty, child-health, and eugenics. However, birth control clinic pioneers were feminists, inspired by the need to confront the problems of women's health, and to 'rescue' contraception from the commercialism of the pharmacy. Marie Stopes' first birth control clinic (1921) was inspired not only by the desire to reduce the physical burden of childbearing on women, but to recognise the fact that sexual pleasure was as much a woman's right as a man's. Initially, birth control clinics were presented as maternity and birth control centres, though legislation on child health (Maternity and Child Welfare Act 1918) which initiated free Government clinics, made the connection redundant.

Thus, the main support the feminists had at this time came from eugenicists and neo-Malthusians interested in the quality of the race, and the economic benefits of population limitation. There was no law in England which could be used to restrict the spread of birth control clinics.

As legal restrictions were virtually non-existent, the dispute over birth control could not be resolved by the courts. The consequence of this was a clash of professional and public opinion which was brought to the attention of the media. This had the effect of bringing sex into open discussion for the first time.

Professional medical opinion was ignorant and instinctively conservative. Physicians considered the birth control movement a moral and physical danger to the community, and had no knowledge of the scientific aspects of contraception.

In 1923, the 'Catholic Confederation' urged the Prime Minister to make voluntary birth control provision illegal. In fact, two Labour (socialist) controlled London boroughs were warned by the Ministry of Health that their funding for maternity services would be withdrawn if they continued to provide contraceptives within these services. In the 1920s, associations were formed to agitate for national provision of birth control clinics. While the Ministry of Health, under pressure from influential Catholics and other reactionaries, prevented welfare centres from giving contraceptive information to mothers, finance from progressive wealthy people permitted the opening of private clinics for birth control. In fact, middle and upper class opinion was more libertarian than working class.

By vote of Parliament (House of Lords) in 1926, the Ministry of Health was permitted to provide finance both for birth control as well as maternity services in public clinics.

By the mid-1930s physicians, Church of England bishops, and the Ministry of Health had all publicly conceded the case for birth control, on the grounds of preventing abortions and reducing the level of maternal mortality (caused by childbearing and illegal abortion). In 1930, all private clinics run by volunteers were amalgamated under the title of the National Birth Control Council - a movement which received political support from political parties of the right, centre and left. (As early as 1910, trade unions and the Labour party had promoted birth control. In 1924, delegates to the Labour Women's Conference formed a Workers' Birth Control Group to unite

- 213 -

women of all movements to bring pressure on Parliament and the male dominated Labour Party to seriously consider contraception and maternal health.)

The new National Birth Control Council (NBCC), subsequently an Association with member branches, urged local authorities to take action under a Ministry of Health memorandum which stated that 'in cases where there are medical grounds for giving advice on contraceptive methods to married women in attendance at the (Maternity and Child Welfare) Clinic, it may be given, but that such advice be limited to cases where a further pregnancy may be detrimental to health, and should be given at a separate session and under conditions such as will not disturb the normal running of the Centre'. The NBCC realised that not all local authorities, were aware of the existence of this Memorandum. Consequently the Ministry of Health eventually was forced to clarify the Memorandum, stating that it had been issued 'solely for the purpose of explaining the views of the Government on the use of institutions controlled by the local authority for the purpose of giving advice to women on contraceptive methods, and it should be understood that the question of providing facilities for giving such advice . . . is entirely a matter within the discretion of the Local Authority'.

During the 1930s, in the period leading up to World War II, political and public opinion turned to a perceived threat of de-population. The term 'birth control' became suspect, and eventually associated with Nazi ideology. Consequently the National Birth Control Association was renamed the Family Planning Association, with emphasis upon promotion of child spacing rather than birth restriction. From this time the FPA emphasised its ability to provide advice on problems of subfertility and sterility.

The volunteer movement for free family planning organised by the FPA collapsed during the war. However, 1945 saw the return of a socialist government committed to the establishment of a free-of-charge comprehensive health care system. Unfortunately, contraception was left out of this formula, being regarded at the time as a luxury. (Moreover, National Health Service physicians knew so little about contraception that they would have been incapable of giving a service at that time.)

The Ministry of Health preferred to continue to avoid the issue of family planning because of the political controversy it still caused through moral/religious objection. Furthermore, it was argued that legislation on the subject was unwarranted as the majority of contraceptors were men using condoms purchased through pharmicists - not women attending clinics.

Confusion over the role of general practitioners in family planning continued through the 1940s. No physician was obliged to give advice unless this was considered necessary for medical treatment. The problem of deciding when birth control advice was 'medical' rather than 'social' was a financial one. The Ministry of Health felt unable to define any circumstances in which treatment would not be medical and where a fee could be charged for such services. Moreover, physicians had little time for or interest in contraception during the post-war years.

Official recognition of the FPA

Official recognition of the FPA was facilitated, in spite of continued opposition, by parliamentary visit by the Minister of Health. When in 1926 a reference had been made to birth control in a BBC radio discussion programme, a spokesman had later apologised, and emphasised that this inadvertent inclusion had not been authorised. In 1955, the Chairman of the FPA, Mrs Margaret Pyke, was able to discuss the work of the Association on the radio without any subsequent apology, and the Times newspaper published a leading article in favour of birth control and praising the FPA.(3)

The oral contraceptive revolution

The rapid rise in popularity of oral contraceptives after 1962 forced the entry of the medical profession into the field in order to supervise the administration of pills. While their involvement was restricted to this method, it was this professional involvement and the enormous demand for the method that led to full statutory provision of free-of-charge contraceptives within the National Health Service.

A number of other factors led to the creation of legislation on planned parenthood which had been fought for for 50 years. The first was the passing of an Abortion Act of the same year as the National Health Service (Family Planning) Act - 1967 (see Issue 6). A Dr Edwin Brooks introduced a private member's bill on family planning enabling local health authorities to provide contraceptive advice, supplies and appliances as part of the NHS. In contrast to the debates on abortion, family planning legislation was relatively uncontroversial, as both MPs and the general public were highly receptive at this time to such social reform.

The National Health Service (Family Planning) Act 1967 gave local health authorities in England and Wales powers to make arrangements for the giving of contraceptive advice and treatment to all who required it, whether on medical or social grounds. Advice and examination were to be free, but a charge could be made for prescription and supply in non-medical cases, at the discretion of the authority.

In monitoring the services, the FPA found that by 1968 difficulties had already arisen from lack of local health authority resources and trained personnel.

The campaign to make family planning services totally free-of-charge within the NHS was signficantly helped in the early 1970s by the Population Lobby. This was a pressure group aiming both to alert the British government and public to the impending crisis of world 'overpopulation', and to show that Britain, itself, suffered from excessive population. Pressure groups such as 'Doctors and Overpopulation' and 'Population Countdown' were formed, aiming to educate the public and parliamentarians on population issues. As a charity, the FPA could not legally engage in pressure group activities, and so formed the Birth Control Campaign (1971), the aim of which was to present the case for totally funded provision for birth control.

In 1972, the Government decided that a substantial extension of family planning services would be required if the numbers of unwanted pregnancies were to be reduced. A parliamentary debate ensued over the issue of free contraception which was decided when the Labour Party took office in 1974, announcing total free contraception from that time - the first universally available, free birth control service in Western Europe.(4)

The unmarried/young

Contraceptive provision for the unmarried represented the boldest advance in the 1967 family planning legislation. However, pre-marital advice had always posed a problem for the FPA due to its concern with organisational respectability and national status. In 1964, the Association decided that it would not provide contraception for the unmarried, but would 'encourage provision' for this group. It was left to Helen Brook, an FPA associate, to open a clinic solely for the young unmarried in 1964 (Brook Advisory Centres).

Issue 1 and 2:   Family planning facilities/services

Allen has recently reported on the status of government (NHS) family planning services through interviews with 100 professional staff and 1,000 female clients. One of the main findings of this research was the extent to which the use of family planning methods and services has become a fact of life for the vast majority of women. The proportion of women who were so unmotivated that they would not use or consider methods of services was found to be very limited. Awareness of the existence of family planning services from clinics and GPs and the knowledge that these were freely available were almost universal among the women interviewed in this study:

> There can be little doubt that the integration of the GPs into free family planning service has been very important, not only in tidying up the provision, but also in encouraging GPs to participate fully in offering family planning advice. This report has shown how important the role of the GP is, with nearly 90 per cent of the samples of women who had recently had babies having spoken about family planning to their own GP, and nearly 50 per cent of them currently using GP family planning services. Nearly three-quarters of the married women in both areas studied said they had never spoken to their GPs about family planning. Levels of satisfaction with GPs' family planning service were very high among all the groups of women we interviewed, and it is obviously an increasingly natural action to regard GPs as the first source of advice on family planning matters.(5)

However, she also noted the doubts of health professionals about whether GPs have enough time and expertise to give a fully comprehensive family planning service. Consequently, most believed it essential that a choice of services between clinics and GPs ought to remain. It was also discovered that women used different services at different times of their lives and substantial numbers of women had used both outlets; that is, they were exercising choice.

Insofar as many GPs offer only the pill and do not have either the interest or expertise in family planning which are necessary if a meaningful choice of service is to be offered, Allen recommended that most women should regard their GP as the first person to approach for the pill, while clinics should always be available for those who would not go to their GP under any circumstances, or those whose GPs do not provide the desired method. Moreover, it was suggested that in the future, famly planning clinics should concentrate on contraceptive method problems, should specialise in IUD and cap insertion, and should extend their counselling and advisory role.

Unfortunately, clinics were found to be crowded and people often had to wait a long time to see a doctor, which undoubtedly discouraged women with young children.

Issues 3 and 4: The Sale, distribution and advertisement of contraceptives; the availability/sale of family planning related literature

Initially, there was no legal restriction on the use or manufacture of contraceptives, nor was there any absolute ban on their sale or availability. The sale of contraceptives through vending machines in public places was later prohibited by most local government authorities, through the Local Government Act 1933 (suppression of nuisances) - legislation which sought to prevent pressure sales of items contrary to 'public taste'. The advertising of contraceptives and the dissemination of birth control literature were subject only to the general law of the land: e.g. the Metropolitan Police Act 1839, making it unlawful to expose to public view any profane, indecent or obscene book, drawing or print. There was no legal restriction on the publication of contraceptive information provided this did not contravene the 1857 Obscene Publications Act, under which the early birth control propagandists were prosecuted.(6)

Even after the war, when the FPA had been recognised as an authoritative and respectable body by the medical profession and general public, this organisation continued to face severe difficulties in publicising family planning. Due to pressure from influential politicians and Catholics, the BBC directorate would not allow a broadcast appeal for funds (to finance clinics). Advertisments were also refused. The notion of 'offending public taste' remains a means by which powerful conservative elements within the media can prevent socially useful and politically progressive media advertising or communication.

However, through the activities of leading figures in the religious (Protestant) as well as medical world, public opinion began to shift. TV and radio interest in family planning was achieved following the much-publicised visit to the FPA, in 1955, by the Minister of Health.

In 1959, the BBC broadcast an appeal by the Bishop of Southwark on behalf of the FPA in its 'Week's Good Cause' series. Attempts to prevent this appeal resulted in widespread support for the FPA. In the House of Lords, Lord Chesham, representing the Government, when replying to a question concerning the programme said that 'if we are to be accused of commiting a political 'gaffe' in allowing this broadcast, just think of the colossal weight of opinion which is going to be offended if we do not'. Other speakers urged that, far from the Association appealing for charity, it was for the Government to consider whether the time had not come to give it assistance from public funds.

In 1960, the British Medical Association Council postponed indefinitely the inclusion of an FPA advertisement in its publications. This provoked another strong public reaction, with the FPA again receiving most of the sympathy. The Times said, in a leading article, 'By general recognition of the majority in this country, the FPA has taken its place among the respectable and useful adjuncts of the social services . . . Doctors and laymen who disapprove of its activities have nothing to do with it, but those non-conformists to the generally accepted pattern of public opinion have no business to seek to interfere with their neighbours.'

Contraceptive advertising restrictions in the UK

The problem of communicating birth control information to the public in the UK has continued apace with the development of new forms of media in the 20th century. In the early part of the century, distributors of contraceptives and abortifacients utilised, albeit discreetly, the pages of women's journals.

Smith provides an overview of the trend towards liberalisation:

> The commercial advertising of methods of contraception is steadily becoming more widespread in spite of the lingering pseudo-fastidiousness of the Independent Broadcasting Authority, London Transport and others. Newspapers and magazines regularly carry advertisements for condoms and other non-medical methods. A typical three month media schedule for one sheath manufacturer ranges across **Honey, 19, Hers, Family Life, TV Times** and the **Daily Express**. The Health Education Council's full page spreads on Casanova and modern methods of contraception run in late 1970 and early 1971 can be seen as a major breakthrough for this type of advertising, combining as it did a motivational message with a factual, understandable method table. Advertising for medical methods, different makes of the 'pill' etc. is commonplace in the professional journals.(7)

Unfortunately, what the respective non-governmental bodies controlling public advertising regard as suitable for public consumption shifts according to their decision over what is 'acceptable'. Bodies such as the Code of Advertising Practice Committee and the Advertising Standards Authority, BBC, IBA, etc. are notoriously non-progressive in matters of sexuality, and highly sensitive to conservative minority group opinion, in spite of what the majority of the public would be willing to accept.

Twelve years after the move toward a more receptive attitude to the broadcasting of family planning issues by the authorities referred to above, a charity organisation wishing to advertise the availability of the relatively new postcoital contraception has been refused permission by most news media.

Describing the problems which have arisen over attempts to alert the public to the availability of postcoital contraception, Johnson reports (8) that such advertisements must be submitted to a 'Code of Advertising Practice Committee'- a non-governmental organisation made up of representatives of advertising agencies, which decided on this occasion that the only 'acceptable' advertising for after-sex birth control was to be 'small classified advertisements'.

The Independent Broadcasting Authority (UK commercial television) does not allow contraceptive methods to be advertised on television or radio on the grounds of unsuitability for 'family' audiences (sic). The question of 'offending public taste' continues to be used as the excuse for refusing family planning information/ advertising.

However, family planning clinics are allowed to communicate their services and the Government-funded Health Education Council (HEC) has used several forms of media in the past. It is worth noting that in any event television is too expensive for family planning charities to utilise in a routine way, even if they were permitted to.

Issue 5: Sterilisation

Sterilisation as a method of contraception does not have a separate history from other methods in the 100 year fight for family planning in the UK (see issues 1 and 2). In this respect, sterilisation was as much subject to attack from the Roman Catholic Church - as against the will of God - as other 'mechanical' or medical methods.

In 1934, the Report of the British Departmental Committee on Sterilisation stimulated consideration of the operation on grounds other than eugenic. In Aberdeen, the policy of Sir Dugald Baird and colleagues from 1935 onward was to offer sterilisation to all women who had failed to prevent recurrent pregnancies.

By the time of the 1967 NHS (Family Planning) Act, which empowered local health authorities in England and Wales to give contraceptive advice and supplies as part of the NHS, male and female sterilisation was omitted largely because hospitals (and GPs) were uninvolved at that time.

Sterilisation was available from private charitable institutions for a fee (e.g. Marie Stopes House; Family Planning Association).

In 1971, the Birth Control Campaign (BCC) pressure group was formed to press for a total (incl. sterilisation) free NHS contraceptive service which included men as well as women. The developments which led to the 1972 NHS (Family Planning) Amendment Act are recounted by Leathard thus:

The BCC had chosen vasectomy as a focal starting point in its campaign for free, comprehensive, birth control services. Local authorities had no powers to finance vasectomy operations, although BCC knew of authorities who wished to develop this service. A growing demand for this method of birth control had been demonstrated by the response to recently opened FPA clinics for male sterilisation in Cardiff (1968), West Bromwich, Glasgow and London (1970). The press and public showed increasing interest. While an estimated 30,000 operations were undertaken in 1972 by private clinics and, on medical grounds only, under the NHS, the FPA still had a reported waiting list of 10,000 and BCC was aware of those who wanted vasectomy but could not afford it.

On 26 October 1972, the National Health Service (Family Planning) Amendment Act at last received the royal assent. Local health authorities could now provide vasectomy services on the same basis as contraception services. This was an important extension of local authority powers, especially as the Secretary of State made it clear that the service was to be 'on the rates' and thus free to the individual . . . BCC could claim much credit for the Bill reaching the Statute Book: through its pressure in the Parliamentary lobby and in the drafting of the Bill itself. However, BCC received considerable help from the FPA, the DHSS and the strong public support for this measure of birth control.(9)

In the UK the acceptance of vasectomy is largely due to the promotion of it by the Simon Population Trust, who in 1966 as part of their nationwide 'Sterilisation Project' attempted to build a channel of communication between men and women who on good grounds wanted to be sterilised, and those gynaecologists and surgeons who were prepared to do the operation. The Trust concentrated on vasectomy. It re-established its legality and publicised the operation, which resulted in its acceptance on wider grounds.

The DHSS has advised health authorities: 'Demand for sterilisation, male and female, is increasing, partly because of the increased risk of cardio-vascular disease in older women, and smokers using oral contraceptives. Sterilisation services should be expanded in coordination with the planning of gynaecological services and family planning clinics' (DHSS Planning Guidelines for 1978/1979, Health and Personal Social Services in England HC(78)12). Contraceptive advice and supplies have been provided free-of-charge on request by the NHS since 1974. However, free sterilisations have not been available in all areas. Health authorities have been allowed discretion concerning the type of service provided, making the availability of an operation for other than strictly medical reasons uneven from area to area. The Birth Control Trust calculated an average waiting time of six months or longer for female sterilisation in 19 of the 30 Area Health Authorities (AHA) answering their questions. Only six of the 30 AHAs had an average waiting time of three months or less. The result is that one-third of all young married couples are likely at present to pay for a private service.

Issue 6:   Abortion

The modern law of abortion in England and Wales rests on two sections of the Offences against the Person Act 1861. Section 58 makes it a felony punishable with life imprisonment for anyone, including the woman, unlawfully to procure an abortion. Section 59 makes it a misdemeanor punishable with imprisonment for three years to supply any instrument, poison or 'noxious thing' for an abortion.

As medical knowledge and technique progressed in the latter half of the 19th century, it became the accepted practice to perform the operation if it was thought necessary to save the woman's life.

The Infant Life (Preservation) Act 1929 made it legal to terminate a viable foetus (that is, one of 28 weeks or more) in order to save the woman's life. The situation did not change until Judge Macnaghten summed up the Bourne case of 1938.(10) According to Macnaghten, it was lawful to terminate, not only to save life but also to safeguard the woman's health and to prevent her being, in his words, 'a physical and mental wreck'.

The Abortion Law Reform Association (ALRA) founded by a group of women in 1936, aimed to repeal the existing abortion law in order to free the medical profession from legal restrictions beyond the medical and social. The high level of maternal mortality from illegal abortion, and the ambiguity of existing laws, brought widespread support for the pressure group.

The 1937 Governmental Committee of Inquiry (Birkett Committee) identified the level of illegal abortion and accompanying maternal mortality. It recommended clarification of the law, 'to make it unmistakenly clear that a medical practitioner is acting legally, when in good faith he procures the abortion of a pregrant woman in circumstances which satisfy him that continuance of the pregnancy is likely to endanger her life or seriously to impair her health'.

In 1948 ALRA met to decide how to change legislation - whether to draft a Private Member's Parliamentary Bill (11) and engage in direct political action, or rely upon the creation of precedents in the law courts. In 1948, more cases came to court, of physicians conducting 'illegal' abortions. As in the Bourne case, the judge ruled in favour of the physicians. Such rulings were encouraging to the small body of campaigners in ALRA. In the years following, ALRA turned more to political action, first within the women's organisations, encouraging the passing of resolutions favouring reform, thereafter engaging in parliamentary lobbying: the process by which members of parliament are systematically informed and encouraged to promote the cause of representatives of a pressure group.

The abortion issue was revived in the UK when, in 1951, the Pope re-stated the Church's objection to birth control and artificial insemination. It was also stated that abortion was not justified even to save the life of the mother.

From the early 1960s Catholic opposition to birth control and abortion was greeted with increasing resistance. When the Thalidomide tragedy occurred, an opinion poll discovered that almost 80% of the public was in favour of reforming the law to enable a woman who wished to do so, to have an abortion rather than be compelled to give birth to a seriously malformed child.

The Society for the Protection of the Unborn Child (SPUC) was formed in 1967 of leading Church of England and medical figures. The aim of SPUC was to challenge any attempt to produce a new abortion law which took consideration of the social factors for termination of pregnancy. This organisation held press conferences, public meetings, etc. and organised petitions in which thousands of signatures were collected to display the level of public opposition to abortion law reform.

and during the 1960s a survey of London physicians indicated support for abortion as a safe operation which should be available on the National Health Survey.

Even after the 1967 Abortion Act (12) was passed it was argued that illicit abortions were still being performed by physicians avoiding taxation. Nevertheless, ALRA maintained that further reform of the law (to provide it 'on demand') would have little practical effect. Hindell and Simms conclude:

> Law reform had been necessary to free doctors to act in the best interests of their patients without fear of prosecution. This had been achieved. But it was to misinterpret the function of law reform to suppose it could solve the practical problems now confronting the Health Service. The real problems were now the attitudes of some doctors, the poor utilisation of hospital facilities, and the fear of some abortion patients who hesitated to consult their doctors. Only time, money, efficient administration and education can solve these problems, not further legislation.(13)

The Lane Committee Report 1974 (on the Working of the 1967 Abortion Act) spoke of the unhappiness which the Act had caused to many NHS nurses. Equally many women have been made unhappy by their inability to obtain the NHS abortion to which they were legally entitled and have been forced to turn to the private sector (that is, are forced to pay for them) - or to continue with an unwanted pregnancy. Since the Abortion Act was passed the proportion of abortions performed by the NHS has gradually declined.

In 1970 the NHS carried out 62% of all abortions but by 1980 this had dropped to 47%. Lack of NHS provision is more serious in some parts of the country than in others (as few as 10% of abortions being carried out on the NHS in some areas). Yet other health districts fulfill 90%+ requests for abortions. The cause of such variation may be traced to the attitudes of the gynaecologists who ultimately perform the operations and the nurses who serve them, and the attitude of the referring GP.

It has been argued that the right of conscientious objection lies at the root of poor NHS provision of this service.(14)

Allen described the problem thus:

One of the problems in the abortion services, mentioned in this report, was the fact that so many women regarded consultations with doctors as 'battles'. There was a strong case for counselling to be given by people who were not necessarily going to have to make a judgement on whether to refer to abortion or not, and there was evidence of a need for counselling to be available from sources other than GPs or gynecological out-patients clinics if required. In our view, properly trained family planning clinic doctors, or possibly nurses or social workers, could fulfil this function, and GPs could refer women about whom they had any doubts to a clinic for further counselling. This should never be used as a delaying tactic and speedy referral would be necessary.'(15)

The Birth Control Campaign position is that the conscientious objection clause (section 4) within the Abortion Act is being abused by many physicians. There is no way that a woman seeking advice from her GP on abortion can know what his/her attitude is; nor is there any obligation on the part of physicians to explain how they are interpreting the Act. Consequently, an unscrupulous physician who is against abortion can delay referral or treatment until the pregnancy is too far advanced.

There is evidence to suggest that delays in the performance of legal abortion are also the result of other administrative shortcomings which mask the above factor. A study of late abortions conducted during 1984 by the Royal College of Obstetricians and Gynecologists for the Department of Health, revealed that:

Women who need abortions face serious delays - sometimes of eight weeks or more - between being referred by a doctor and having the operation . . . Deficiencies in health service administration contribute substantially to the hold-ups . . . One in five of the women who had the operation between 20 and 23 weeks gestation had been referred by doctors before the end of the 12th week . . . yet they faced delays at this critical time of eight weeks or more . . . Nearly 40 per cent of those who had abortions at 15-16 weeks had been referred by their local doctors before the 12th week; they had to wait for three weeks or more.

Young women fared worst - women under 20 accounted for more than 40 per cent of the late abortions, and more than 50 per cent of the very late abortions. Significantly, more than one in five of the women having very late abortions had been refused the operation in previous pregnancies.

The vast majority of women needing late abortions turn to the private sector: a ratio of six to one with the NHS. Delays in the private sector are less frequent.(16)

A survey of abortion provision in one Regional Health Authority (17) suggests that hospital gynaecologists present a greater problem to the client than the referring GP. Ashton found that 12 of the 32 NHS gynaecologists there expressed conscientious objections to abortion and were directly responsible for delays which forced women to turn to the private sector.

Recommendations presented by the Birth Control Campaign to resolve problems in the functioning of the Abortion Act include the following:

Firstly, **day-care services,** which have been shown to be acceptable to the women involved; the abortion is carried out earlier in the pregnancy which is safer for the woman and pleasanter for the staff: only staff who have no reservations about abortion treatment need to be involved. A day-care abortion unit can be completely separate from other gynecological services, while retaining the necessary theatre back-up facilities and it is considerably cheaper to run than the equivalent in-patient service, an important factor in times of financial stringency. Unfortunately, the NHS has failed to establish the necessary units.

Secondly, where the NHS is unwilling or unable to provide an abortion service then consideration can be given to **contracting out** the abortion service to one of the two abortion charities (which has already been done in some parts of Britain). This is believed to have the following advantages: the service is run by experienced professionals; the staff choose to work in this specialist area; the service is geared to the needs of the woman; and the counselling is built into the system in a way rarely found in NHS provision.

Thirdly, it is argued that greater understanding is necessary among nurses of the need for abortion services; that is, to involve nurses and midwives in the discussions and consultations on abortion which take place both in the community and in hospital, enabling those working in the community to see for themselves the patient and family environment:

'There may perhaps be a need for more general support and counselling of nurses to help them come to terms with many of the difficulties they encounter in their day-to-day work'.(18)

Fourthly, 'it would be helpful if women wanting an abortion knew what the attitude of their GP was (and therefore) it should be possible to devise a method for ensuring that those GPs who have a conscientious objection to abortion register this objection publicly, for example by indicating this in the Medical List published by local Family Practitioner Committees and available in public libraries. This would avoid much distress - to woman and doctor alike - and remove some of the 'hurdle' aspect to discussions about abortion'.(19)

Issue 7: Infertility Treatment

See National Profile and Recommendations.

Issue 8: Sex education/family life education

Placed in historical perspective, the controversial issue of school sex education provision may be traced to social changes which began a century ago in the economic conditions of families, in child mortality rates and in formal education. As Weeks contends, attitudes to sexuality over the last two centuries must be related to changes in the socio-economic sphere. In the context of capitalist society where the family was being transformed in line with new property relations (wife and children as extensions of 'private property'), it is suggested that sexuality operated and was seen as a threat to this power relationship.(20)

A reduction in family size had resulted from increased chances of survival of offspring. The provision of state education, moreover, increased the dependency of (non-employed) children on their parents. Weeks describes the social-psychological consequence of this as two-fold: 'an increased emotional investment in each child' and 'a shift of concern by the male power-holder from the sexual power of the female to that of the adolescent' (21) . The resulting family tensions were fed by and provided the seed for an independent youth 'culture' with its own courting rituals.

Contemporary anxieties about sex education in schools, however distorted or amplified by certain media, can be partly explained by reference to this 19th century objection by parents to an unprecedented loss of control over their children following the introduction of compulsory elementary education after 1870. Where school sex education exists, research suggests that it promotes values which most parents would accept (general respect for married life, personal hygiene, etc.).(22) However, such knowledge, given to young people independently of parents, is still (consciously or sub-consciously) a source of apprehension. The potential use made of 'taboo' knowledge by adolescents to reinforce and extend their age/cultural independence merely confirms the subversive role of sex education of any kind which is not under the control of/imparted by parents.

This continuing lack of confidence in the ascribed purpose of 'formal' sex education is unfortunately not resolved by the 'scandal' of teenage pregnancy and abortion rates, whose link with sex education is made according to the persuasion or prejudice of those concerned rather than any scientific correlation.

However positive the response of governments to authorise sex education in schools - whatever the content - the British educational system does not readily permit the standardisation of curricula in any sphere, least of all sex education. Burke describes the situation thus:

> The structure of the education system is such that specific activities in a particular school are left to the discretion of the head teacher of that school, who is expected to adjust recommendations from Central and Local Government to suit the needs of his own school community. As a result of the autonomous organisation of each school, there is wide diversity in sex education activities, as in many other spheres, in different parts of the country. However,

each school is answerable to a Local Education Authority, which in some instances attempts to influence the head teachers of the schools of its area by producing reports and circulating recommendations. There are 163 Local Education Authorities in England and Wales. Each of these is responsible to the Central Government, and is expected to promote national education policies at the local level, as well as undertaking general administrative functions in the organisation and co-ordination of the educational institutions in a particular area.(23)

However well meaning the recommendations of all of these bodies, it remains unclear how <u>effective</u> the content of sex education is in those schools willing to teach the subject. For the problem is not so much 'whether' but 'how far' sex education should be the responsibility of schools or parents. The 1980s are in many ways a reaction to the liberal ideas of the 1960s and 1970s. Attempts to further the cause of progressive sex education are resisted by a reactionary press and parliamentary representatives of right-wing moral pressure groups.

Provision of school sex education in Britain displays the following characteristics according, to Kozakiewicz and Rea(24):

There is no centrally elaborated and compulsory sex education curriculum for schools . . . there are no obligatory textbooks on sex education, although a great variety are available (this relates to the autonomy of the teacher in British education). The same is true of teachers' handbooks. It was generally felt that the supply of books and all kinds of audio/visual and textural materials was poor, but occasionally sufficient; schools make use of special broadcasts on educational television.

There is some special sex education training for teachers (in some colleges or departments) during basic training or post-experience training, and special sex education courses are available for all kinds of professional workers - teachers, physicians, priests, health visitors etc. On the whole, it is teachers who deal with sex education in schools, but health education officers, medical officers, nurses, members of the PPA and the Marriage Guidance Council also play an important role in some schools. There are no obligatory courses to prepare teachers for sex education, but about 10% of teachers' colleges have optional courses to which approximately 16 hours per annum are devoted. It should be noted that in the British system there is a network of Teachers' Centres, Curriculum Development Centres etc. which may promote on a small local basis courses for teachers in that locality.

In the United Kingdom, the content of sex education is rarely discussed professionally or publicly, let alone decided upon nationally. Consequently, the subject remains fixed at a stage where details are contested by a number of competing pressure groups and authorities. Much interest in the subject - particularly by the mass media - is less than responsible.

It is understandable, therefore, that Government remains aloof from the discussions and has never legislated on the subject other than in peripheral ways (see below). The only issue which has forced government involvement in the subject in the past has been that of increasing teenage pregnancy - where money has been spent on piecemeal publicity campaigns aimed to discourage the young from early intercourse. Predictably, such efforts have been strongly criticised for different reasons from both right and left.

The extract below is taken from the most recent Government statement on the subject of sex/health education in schools. As a Government document purporting to provide 'guidelines', this is significant both in the cautiousness of its pronouncements, its lack of specificity and its side-stepping of the problem of retaining some standardised teaching curriculum in this field in the face of open invitation to parents to challenge any item within it:

Health education, like preparation for parenthood, is part of the preparation of the individual for personal, social and family responsibilities. Health education should give pupils a basic knowledge and understanding of health matters both as they affect themselves and as they affect others, so that they are helped to make informed choices in their daily lives. It should also help them to become aware of those moral issues and value judgements which are inseparable from such choices. Preparation for parenthood and family life should help pupils to recognise the importance of those human relationships which sustain, and are sustained by, family life, and the demands and duties that fall on parents.

Schools are responding in a variety of ways to the need for sound sex education. Sex education is one of the most sensitive parts of broad programmes of health education, and the fullest consultation and cooperation with parents are necessary before it is embarked upon. In this area offence can be given if a school is not aware of, and sensitive to, the cultural background of every child. Sex education is not a simple matter and is linked with attitudes and behaviour. The regulations to be made under Section 8 of the Education Act 1980 will require Local Education Authorities (LEAs) to inform parents of the ways and contexts in which sex education is provided.(25)

Issue 9: Adoption

See national profile.

PPA recommendations to government

A Service - General Secretary UKFPA

General

Most restrictions on the exercise of planned parenthood as a human right in the United Kingdom can be traced to one of four causes:

- Restrictions on expenditure by the National Health Service and the state education system.

- The opposition by influential minorities to fertility regulation in general and to provision of education and facilities to young people in particular.

- Resistance to change by the educational and medical professions.

- Ambivalence in the media and advertising professions, leading to titillation and sensationalising of sexuality in media coverage and advertisements, but refusal of advertising aiming to increase effective fertility control.

Most of the recommendations given below have to face and overcome one or more of these four obstacles if the desired human right is to be available in reality.

Issue 1:   Family planning facilities/services

Government in the UK, regardless of political party, has a strong commitment to free planned parenthood services, based on legislation of the 1970s. The first major government action needed regarding family planning services is clear direction to health authorities that the availability of choice outlet between General Practitioners (60 per cent of users) must be fully maintained, for this choice is under threat in the current search for financial savings.

The second major action needed by government is an initiative to make family planning services more available to the male partners of sexual relationships, by recommending health authorities to encourage their doctors and other professionals, by providing relevant training, and by permitting General Practitioners to prescribe condoms.

A third need is for encouragement of wider knowledge and use of post-coital birth control among doctors and the public.

Issue 2:   Services for young people

Most (66 per cent) of the roughly 200,000 unplanned pregnancies in the UK each year occur to those in the 16-25 year old group. Yet of the over 200 health authorities, only 60 provide youth advisory services and a further 15 contract Brook Advisory Centres to give the special facilities that young people need if they are to use family planning services. Government guidance to health authorities on the basis of research and pilot projects, is much needed.

Issue 3:   Sale, distribution and advertising of contraceptives

Government has recently assisted planned parenthood organisations in persuading the Independent Broadcasting Authority to permit regional television stations to broadcast UK FPA and Brook 30-second Public Service Announcements (free-of-charge) on young men's responsibility in sex and contraception, and eight TV channels are now doing this with hardly a sign of public protest. Research has shown, however, that advertising naming brands of products is necessary to show really good results in public take-up. Government should therefore assist with further negotiations to ensure effective press and media advertising and should encourage further advertising in this field of health by the Health Education Council.

Issue 4:   Planned parenthood literature

The UK has a Government-funded service of family planning information literature, run by the UK FPA, that is notable in scale by the standards of other countries. The major restrictions on it, apart from financial limitations in relation to public demand, are on the relevance of the language employed in leaflets to those most in need of information. Government should wherever possible allow the use of vernacular language and clear illustrations, accepting that these attract criticism from minorities who oppose family planning. Government should also encourage the use of new outlets that will communicate with parts of the community not in touch with conventional NHS services.

Issue 5:   Sterilisation services

Sterilisation, where desired, is a highly cost-effective and satisfactory method of contraception. Government should therefore advise those health authorities not providing adequate sterilisation facilities for public demand to increase their provision on the basis of health and economic research.

Issue 6:   Abortion services

In the foreseeable future, abortion will continue to be a necessary back-up service for people who have not used contraception successfully and whose pregnancy should not continue.

Government action is needed firstly to ensure that early day-care abortion, known to be extremely desirable and cost-effective yet still available in only some 20 NHS units in the UK, becomes available as a norm among health authorities. Secondly, health authorities should be advised to provide in-service training for relevant staff on attitudes to abortion, to encourage understanding and reduce the hostility often met by abortion patients. Thirdly, GPs should be reminded that if they have personal objections to abortion, they should inform relevant patients and advise them to see another doctor. Fourthly, health authorities unwilling for any reason to provide abortion should be reminded by government that there are two major reputable abortion charities to whom authorities can contract out.

Issue 7:   Infertility services

Sub-fertility and infertility services are provided by the National Health Service, but as with sterilisation and abortion the provision by health authorities is very uneven. In some areas, especially where there are teaching hospitals, public needs are well met. In most parts of the country, however, waiting lists are long. The National Association for the Childless has recently established an offshoot charity, the Childless Trust, which is hoping to build up a network of private centres to cater for the need unmet by the NHS. Government is now considering the Warnock Committee Report on Human Reproduction and Embryology, and it is hoped that this will result in recommendations on NHS provision as well as guidelines for practice.

Issue 8:   Sex education

Given the control of curriculum by individual schools (rather than by government policy) in Britain, it is difficult to recommend realistic action by Government. It is understood that in liaison committees between the Department of Health and the Department of Education, the health needs of young people for education on sex and planned parenthood are frequently urged. The Department of Education has moved cautiously to encourage schools to provide this in the context of Health Education, but little has been heard since the 1981 School Curriculum document was published. Schools are required since that time to notify the Department of Education about their sex education programmes, and the DHSS might best pursue the matter by asking for a progress report and then suggesting next steps.

REFERENCES

1. Steadman-Jones, G. Outcast London 1971 Peregrine, London.

2. See Meredith, P. Pharmacy, Contraception and the Health Care Role 1982 FPA, London.

3. Information Factsheet 1983 FPA London.

4. GPs were to be brought into the service, with payments for fitting IUDs and prescribing pills. For these there would be no prescription charge. However, GPs refused to provide free condoms for men, as they were regarded as 'non-medical devices'.

5. Allen, I. Family Planning, Abortion and Sterilisation Services 1981 Policy Studies Institute, London.

6. For an account of the pioneering role of the pharmacist in the dissemination of contraceptive information and supplies in 19th and 20th century Britain see Meredith, P. 1982 op cit Ch 1.

7. Smith, W. Campaigning for Choice 1978 FPA p. 7.

8. Johnson, T, Postcoital Contraception Pregnancy Advisory Services 1982 pp. 54-55.

9. Leathard, A. The Fight for Family Planning 1980 p. 190.

10. The legal case concerned a 14 year old schoolgirl raped and made pregnant by soldiers in 1938. Whereas a Roman Catholic gynaecologist refused to abort the pregnancy, Mr Bourne, a consultant obstetrician, agreed to do this having satisfied himself that she was emotionally disturbed by the incident. He was taken to court and tried but acquitted on the grounds that it was impossible to distinguish between a woman's life being in danger and her health being in danger. Due to ambiguity and indecision within the law and the medical profession, in establishing the health grounds for abortion, the Bourne judgement liberalised the abortion law - in practice. The decision was heavily criticised, particularly by Roman Catholics (though Bourne received more public support than condemnation). Bourne had initially agreed to perform the abortion because of a request from the newly-formed Abortion Law reform Association.

11. Such action refers to the use of the Private Member's Bill to achieve changes in legislation which would not be undertaken by the party in power at the time. Until the 19th century, all of the time of the House of Commons

was open to all elected Members of Parliament to propose Bills unconnected with Ministerial legislation. During the 20th century, private member's bill time has been limited. Although it has been argued that private members should not legislate at all, as only governments have the necessary authority to deal with a subject properly, since the 1950s, private member's bills have been powerful means to changing laws such as those relating to obscenity, homosexuality, capital punishment, family planning and divorce. This is an important aspect of parliamentary democracy where the government in power is unwilling to take action on specific social issues. Unfortunately, the restrictions surrounding private member's bills: the limited time for discussion (where a bill can 'fail' because of lack of time) and the fact that there is great competition for such presentations (six members' bills were chosen, by chance, out of 200 at the time of the 1967 Act), makes this a less than perfect method of law making.

12. The Abortion Act provided that a person should not be guilty of an offence when a pregnancy was terminated by a registered medical practitioner if two registered medical practitioners were of the opinion, formed in good faith, that the continuance of the pregnancy would involve risk to the woman's life or injury to the physical or mental health of herself or any existing children of her family, greater than if the pregnancy were terminated. The Act said quite plainly that in determining an abortion 'account may be taken of the pregnant woman's actual or foreseeable environment'.

13. Hindell, D. & Simms, M. Abortion Law Reformed 1971 Peter Owen, London p. 224.

14. Abortion and Conscientious Objection 1983 Birth Control Campaign London.

15. Allen, I. 1981 op cit p. 117.

16. Guardian newspaper report 1984 London.

17. Lancet 19 January 1980.

18. Op cit pg 12.

19. Op cit pg 12.

20. Weeks, J. Sex, Politics and Society 1981 Longman, London.

21. Op cit p. 73.

22. Weeks, J. 1981 op cit Longman, London.

23. Sue Burke (ed) Responsible Parenthood and Sex Education 1970 IPPF, London.

24.   Rea, N. and Kozakiewicz, M. A Survey on the Status of Sex Education in European Member Countries 1975 IPPF Europe p. 40.

25.   The School Curriculum 1981 Department of Education and Science, Her Majesty's Stationary Office March 1981 p. 7f.

History of the Development of Planned Parenthood as a Basic Human Right in Yugoslavia
N Petric

Organised family planning began in Yugoslavia in the 1930s due to the influx of women into industrial occupations demanding birth control. The family planning movement was also a consequence of greater educational standards and the work of the early socialist movements.

The need for effective means of family spacing became more acute following World War II due to the extensive involvement of women, both in industry and in socio-political life. The principal source of progressive views in this area was the Commission for Women within the Yugoslav Trade Union Confederation's Central Council. This Commission, along with other organisations, worked to change laws governing planned parenthood and to promote the practice of family planning as a basis for female emancipation.

In 1961, the Women's Movement in Yugoslavia formed the organisational basis for the creation of Family Planning Council of Yugoslavia (FPCY) in 1963. The broad task of this campaigning and educational body was to be 'the humanisation of relations between the sexes'. The narrow task was to promote responsible parenthood, that is the birth of wanted children.

In 1969 the Council's work was given formal recognition at the Federal level through the Federal Assembly Resolution on Family Planning. This Resolution identified the socio-political function as well as the social, educational, and health aspects of planned parenthood.

As a consequence of the Resolution, the notions of responsible parenthood and humanisation of relations between the sexes were made integral components of the educational curricula for young people, and promoted among the adult population through the media. The Federal legal regulation of planned parenthood was subsequently applied to the municipalities. The inclusion of free decision-making on childbearing into the Constitution was achieved through public discussion and referendum which designated planned parenthood as a human right.

This right to free choice on childbearing, as enshrined within 1974 Federal, Republican and Provincial Constitutions, also entails a duty to fulfill the role of parenthood responsibly, though without enforcing the raising of children solely within the natural parental family circle. The general principles of the 1974 Constitution may be adjusted however to the different conditions pertaining in different communities.

In 1978, the Federal Assembly, in response to female unemployment, particularly in the less developed regions, adopted a Resolution to promote the role of women. This Resolution points out: 'While adopting mid- and long-term plans, we must have in mind demographic trends and their influence on overall trends . . . since childbearing and parenthood are of the broadest social interest, it is both the family and society that have to protect motherhood and the accomplishment of parenthood'.

In 1984, the main task in securing family planning as a human right is the creation of the social conditions necessary for this right to become a practical possibility. To this end, the FPCY has undertaken scientific projects with the assistance of the United Nations Fund for Population Activities (UNFPA). Such projects include an investigation of training facilities for sex and contraceptive educators. Problems lie not so much with availability of contraceptives, as in information and education for the general population - a problem of traditional practices and attitudes.

Transformation of the family

After 1945, the traditional patriarchal family began to undergo transformation, largely due to increasing female employment and consequent economic independence, but also through the participation of women in the liberation struggle. After 1946, the Constitution and laws regulating marriage, relations between parents and children, guardianship and adoption, put family relations on a new basis, proclaiming the protection of marriage and the family to be of special public concern. Church jurisdiction was abolished and monogamy enforced (previously polygamy was permitted to Muslims). Full equality between men and women in marital and family relations, divorce, and in respect of children, was decreed. Where it was previously an institution designed to perpetuate the family line, adoption was now permitted to 'ensure the welfare of orphans'. While new legislation has paved the way for new relationships, problems in these new relationships have also created the need for further legislation to resolve socio-economic problems.

Family planning, population policy and demographic trends in the Socialist Federal Republic of Yugoslavia

In Yugoslavia people cannot realise their human rights as isolated and 'private' beings - but only socially, by collectively changing the overall conditions of their work and life. Similarly, problems of biological reproduction cannot be treated separately from other social relations. The role of both sexes as equal participants in society's productive process and management, not only transforms social but also sexual relationships. In Yugoslav society, based on the principle of self-management, it is possible to overcome the conflict between the individual right to free and responsible parenthood on the one hand, and national population policy on the other, through a constant harmonisation of both interests. Thus, the different demographic trends in the republics and provinces of Yugoslavia do not justify permitting greater free choice in childbearing to one couple in one region vis-à-vis another.

Population policy is being increasingly regarded as a component of a broader socio-economic policy: where development of material resources goes hand in hand with fertility regulation. During the 20th century two significant developments have had a large impact on demographic trends - higher average life expectancy and contraception.

This 'demographic' transition which took place in the second half of the 19th century and during the 20th century, has had important socio-economic consequences. Yugoslavia can be said to represent the world in miniature with respect to its demographic transition. By the 1981 census, there were 22,428,000 inhabitants.

Although this is the largest population of nations on Yugoslavian territory in history, it is noted that in some regions, for example Croatia and Vojvodina, the population increase is low, in contrast with Kosovo, where the birthrate is one of the highest in Europe.

The reasons for the fall in mortality rates have been attributed to the development of modern medicine. By contrast, fertility decline is first and foremost a consequence of socio-economic change - only when a certain level of development is reached does a population become increasingly conscious of the need to adjust life-style and family size. However, it is also true that certain population trends can also influence overall socio-economic development.

Planned parenthood as a basic human right developed in response to the need for the social system to help people manage their biological reproduction and to adjust relations between the sexes to modern socio-economic developments. Several fields have been developed with the aim of implementing this right:

Education: Education in Yugoslavia is based on the achievements of modern science, especially Marxism, in the form of scientific socialism. It aims at preparing people for work and self-management in the spirit of the socialist revolution, ethics, self-management and democracy. The fundamental approach to family planning in Yugoslav society stems from the belief that people must be given the conditions and have access to knowledge to better affect their mutual relations in the intimate sphere, and to be better prepared for free and responsible decision-making on childbearing. Education in human relations between the sexes is considered an integral part of general social education.

Certain republics and provinces have organised seminars with teachers, using a multidisciplinary approach with great success. The Yugoslav People's Army also began organising activities in this field aimed at young people undertaking military service.

The need for special approaches to youth and adults has given rise to extra-curricular institutions known as 'schools for life' and 'schools for parents'. The former are provided in youth and adult education centres. The programme is composed of preparation for professional life, preparation for life in society and preparation for marriage and family.

Scientific research work: The FPCY has developed cooperation with the United Nations Fund for Population Activities. Since 1977 seven projects have been undertaken covering social policy, family planning, medicine, demography (problems in underdeveloped areas in Macedonia) and education (for social workers). Postgraduate studies have been organised for experts in various fields. In preparation are projects on marital and premarital counselling, and concerning the role of the mass media in population and family planning education.

The mass media: The mass media present positive social trends relating to women's social status and have often been one step ahead of practice in the field of family planning. The media play a major role in disseminating knowledge on the advantages and possibilities of preventing undesired pregnancy, and the availability of abortion. The women's and youth press have played a particularly important role in popularising family planning, countering conservative ideas and attacks from the Catholic Church. Periodicals offer concrete information on obtaining contraception and counselling services, answering questions and influencing opinions.

The daily press has also undertaken polls on family planning via health education experts. It has a positive role in spreading scientific knowledge on family planning and sex in general as well as condemning reactionary ideas.

Specially made films for family planning have been little used for education purposes. Several short films have been made but they have been given insufficient publicity. Compared with the earlier taboo on sex in the information media, today certain periodicals have gone to the other extreme, exaggerating sexuality as a major personal and social question. There is also a tendency towards commercialisation of sex which continues the oppression of women.

Taken as a whole, the information media, especially radio and television, have become increasingly involved in family planning; for example, several television programmes devoted to problems were well received by audiences in Slovenia, Serbia, Macedonia and elsewhere. In 1971 and 1972 Slovenia introduced an experimental TV programme geared to parents and youth prepared in cooperation with British television. A survey was conducted to explore public attitudes to this sex education programme. In answer to the question who should handle sex education, the following replies were given: schools 83%, families 82%, television 56%, literature 52%, film 38%. Numerous manuals have also been printed for school teaching in this field.

Case Study: Yugoslavia

Family planning facilities/services

Since 1974, when the human right to planned parenthood became a Constitutional right, the corresponding legal provisions were adopted by republics and provinces to integrate all necessary services. Thus, all family planning services are included in a minimum health protection for all citizens. Respective health institutions were authorised and empowered to provide family planning services including counselling (GP as well as gynecological clinics). Private clinics do not exist. Family planning is also given increasing attention in the work programmes of socio-political organisations and institutions working in the field of health education (e.g. Socialist Alliance, Trade Union Confederation, Union of Socialist Youth, Red Cross, adult education centres, schools, local communities etc.).

Hormonal contraceptives and IUDs are free of charge as are other medicaments and are available with a prescription. Other devices can be bought in pharmacies or other places. There are few manufacturers of contraceptives, but their import is not restricted. In spite of the network of family planning services insufficient numbers of couples resort to contraception, particularly in rural areas.

Abortion

Even before World War II, abortion was a widespread method of regulating childbirth. According to the estimates of medical experts, 50 years ago there were about 300,000 abortions a year, only 50,000 of which were performed legally in health institutions for reasons of health. Because of the severe medical consequences of unskilled abortions, especially among the poorer strata of the population, progressive forces called for abortion to be made accessible to all women.

Today, abortion is legal in all the republics and provinces and is permitted on request, up to 10 weeks gestation, providing there is no risk to health. Abortion after 10 weeks is permitted on request by special commission. If the first application is refused, an appeal may be forwarded to a higher commission.

For adolescents and minors there are special conditions: the parents or guardians have to be informed and have to give their consent to the abortion.

In spite of well-organised family planning services (contraception and information), abortion in Yugoslavia is still widespread. According to approximate data in 1983 there have been about 336,102 abortions, i.e. 87.9 per 100 live births. Illegal abortion is practically non-existent. A decline in the number of abortions since 1967 is believed to be the result of improvement of health/family planning services in spreading contraception, as a wider choice of contraceptives has been made available.

According to a recently published poll on the 'Fertility of Married Women and Family Planning', undertaken by the Centre for Demographic Research, married couples want to plan their families without the involvement of health and social services. This poll showed that 78% of married women are against unplanned pregnancy and that 65% of women in urban areas and 50% of women in rural areas use 'traditional' methods of contraception due to lack of modern methods, which result in numerous abortions and abandoned babies and children. The majority of married couples plan their families without contacting health institutions. They used the following contraceptive methods: orals 8.6%; IUDs 2%; condoms, diaphragms and chemical devices 4.5%; coitus interruptus 79%; others 5.9%.

Increased knowledge of contraceptive methods is hindered by an insufficiently developed network of health institutions in rural areas and in some underdeveloped regions.

The health care of mother and child is of major concern to the health services in Yugoslavia. It is carried out through health centres, general practitioners, specialised health institutions such as clinics for women, students, etc.

From 1955, certain health institutions in the republic and provincial centres have made an important contribution to increase knowledge of contraceptive methods, thereby preventing abortions, and undertaken research into sterility. Some health institutions have established special departments for sterilisation and infertility treatment.

It is possible to see elements of Yugoslavia's selective pronatalist policy in its programme for infertility treatment, longer postpartum leave of absence from the workplace, and other assistance for large families. This includes, in the Vojvodina region in particular, assistance to unemployed young women to provide the means for them to marry and bear children while seeking employment. The fertility rate in this part of the country is very low and the abortion rate very high. The reason stems from desire for small families, though divorce is also an element - being particularly high. One in four marriages end in divorce within five years, 50% without children. Nevertheless, there is also a very low take-up of family planning practices. The preference for abortion over contraception has never been successfully explained from a sociological/psychological point of view.

The Constitution gives the right to individuals to have as well as prevent births. Thus infertility treatment is promoted (12.7% of married women, widows and divorced women remain without children). Infertility treatment in Vojvodina aims to help 30,000 married women between 20-39 who are without children.

Contribution of the Socialist Federal Republic of Yugoslavia to international recognition of family planning as a basic human right

The late President Josip Broz-Tito was among the 12 signatories of the Declaration of World Leaders on family planning as a basic human right. He pointed out that family planning constituted an integral part of the economic development of any country, and that it is necessary for the whole international community to help developing countries overcome difficulties in their socio-economic development. The population issue must be approached in the same way. As the President noted in a letter to John Rockefeller III (reiterated in the message to the World Conference held in Bucharest in 1974), 'then more incentives and realistic preconditions might evolve conducive to changing attitudes to family planning'.

Obstacles to planned parenthood as a basic human right

The school curriculum includes the teaching of responsible parenthood and the improvement of human relations. Teachers are not well trained in this subject. Also, conservatism and traditionalism impede the teaching and acceptance of such a programme, and a shortage of contraceptives means an increase in the number of abortions.

Premarital and marital counselling centres are important to the development of women. These centres influence the population's reproductive behaviour and the status of women.

Since biological reproduction is an integral part of social reproduction in our society, working people are being forced by social conditions to take more responsibility regarding planning a family. Families are the responsibility not only of parents but other members of the community. Therefore, family planning is provided for in the Constitution, as is free decision-making on childbearing in a socially responsible way.

The modern notion of family planning as a basic human right is characterised by the increasingly important role of the family, not marriage. The family is no longer formed on the basis of wedlock, but because of a baby, or adopted child, or because of other lasting forms of care for the child, with the child as the central figure in the family. Family legislation in republics and provinces is based on a unique ideological and political approach, i.e. the full equality and rights of parents, namely parents in all spheres of life, including the human right to decide freely on childbirth.

Chapter Seven

CONCLUSION

Postscript: The Dubrovnik Seminar

This report has presented a comparison of current laws relating to planned parenthood in 18 countries with the quality of services to which these laws relate. This has provided a means to make a crude comparison of the extent to which planned parenthood has been awarded the status of a 'right' similar to that accorded, for example, education or health. It also stands as a measure of the sincerity or commitment of European governments to upholding the right to the number and spacing of children enshrined in international declarations to which they are signatories.

The 18 national profiles have revealed, with small exception, a recently attained high degree of convergence in legislation - displaying a decisive break with the past and a recognition of public demands in this sphere.

The secondary focus of this project was upon the willingness of principally state health systems to respond positively to the liberal, 'enabling' planned parenthood legislation created over the last 50 years, by providing the necessary clinical and administrative resources.

However, these de facto situations revealed a greater degree of variation vis-à-vis law, though with common obstacles to implementation of laws. Nevertheless, countries with quite different cultural and political backgrounds possess similar strengths and weaknesses due to the problems presented by the issues themselves. Thus, there is greatest uniformity, both de jure and de facto, in both the absence of legal restrictions on, for example, the availability of family planning related literature (with the exception of Ireland); on the sale, advertisement and distribution of non-medical contraceptives; and in the presence of protective legislation covering the health and safety of medical contraceptives.

Although not always legally recognised as such, it appears that sterilisation is practiced as a method of family planning in all countries without explicit objection at government level. It is anomalous, therefore, that quite unrelated laws concerning bodily mutilation should in so many countries have a deterrent effect on both the provision and use made of this contraceptive method. It is open to question whether legislation offers an appropriate route to resolving this situation.

On the subject of abortion, it appears that laws are carefully formulated both to define eligibility and to identify their intention. In several countries, the role of abortion as a means of protecting the family unit as well as the health of the mother is explicitly stated. Problems of the exercise of rights which these laws confer largely stem from the grey area of conscientious objection of the health personnel involved.

The absence of legislation on the treatment of infertility (other than that which protects the rights of children born thereof) is likely to be due in part to the lack of public/media attention given to this until recent years. However, it is curious that so little government attention is paid to its promotion in view of the increasing European concern with long-term fertility decline.

The findings on sex and family life education largely reveal non-existent or ineffective legislation, and common weaknesses at the de facto level. Here there appears to be a reluctance and inability on the part of educational authorities to enable/oblige teachers to fulfil recommendations or follow directives. A universal obstacle to the effective implementation of law/recommendation in this sphere stems partly from lack of standardised curricula and pedagogical materials (sanctioned by teachers and the public), and (by implication) the means necessary to train teachers. This contrasts with the reported adequacy of family planning related materials available.

For a variety of controversial reasons, adolescents suffer disproportionately from a lack of services, information and education appropriate to their situations. With the possible exception of Sweden and Denmark, there is a notable reluctance of governments to compromise their positions by entering the subject of the rights as well as the responsibilities of the (unmarried) young in the area of sexuality and contraception.

The countries examined in depth revealed that the level of governments' involvement in aspects of planned parenthood is more a measure of the need to fulfil their own demographic objectives or to react to the demands of pro- or anti-family planning pressure groups, than to unilaterally offer their populations the right to control their fertility. It is important that the PPA, as a primary pressure group in this field, develop the means of presenting the planned parenthood case in a way which identifies how government will also benefit from supporting this case.

The question of improving the relationship between PPA and government, was the subject of a two day seminar convened by the IPPF Europe Region in Dubrovnik, Yugoslavia, December 1984. This seminar provided a forum for selected individuals working within 8 national government departments, and their counterparts in 9 national PPAs, to exchange views on the findings of this project and the PPA recommendations which concluded the case studies.

Postscript: The Dubrovnik Seminar

This seminar* was not based on the assumption that solutions to problems of planned parenthood rights could or should always and only be found in government action, but to discuss the issue: what can be realistically expected of governments as law-makers/administrators (as opposed to organisations such as the medical profession) in the light of their broader responsibilities to society and to their electorate?

The commentary following focusses on a selection of themes which generated discussion among the participants:

1. What are the costs and benefits of establishing close working relations between a PPA and its respective government department dealing with planned parenthood affairs? What strategies can be adopted to improve this relationship?

Despite their endorsement of international declarations on the right of individuals to decide on the number and spacing of children, nations often adopt a different 'national consciousness' of these affairs in deciding what may and may not be regarded as a right.

*See Appendix 2: Dubrovnik Seminar List of Participants (p. 273f).

Thus, the French PPA case study reports that although the French government has not wanted to refuse to acknowledge the existence of this right, abortion is still part of the penal code. Equally, by understanding family planning to refer only to reversible contraceptive methods, 'France can sign declarations with a clear conscience while still failing to offer men and women the same choices as other countries' (p. 186). Although abortion is generally available to the population in Britain, the law does not give any woman the right to abortion, but is concerned only with the circumstances in which a physician carrying out a termination of pregnancy will not be subject to criminal prosecution. The same applies to other dimensions of planned parenthood.

It was noted that it is for the PPA to endeavour to secure government support for practical initiatives in planned parenthood rather than simply moral support for its principles. As a government invariably stands between opposing sectional interests of pressure groups on whose support it relies to remain in power, it will rely on the non-governmental sector to present initiatives. Unfortunately, this is fraught with the often politically negative implication of tying both government and PPA down to a particular ideological standpoint which will generate critical reaction from other sectors of the community. Many countries represented have governments which operate under the influence and scrutiny of powerful conservative political groups. The PPA, itself, risks disintegration of a wide political spectrum of support in attempts to concretise recommendations on the realisation of planned parenthood needs/rights.

The problems of defining a national curriculum for sex education reveal the stalemate ensuing from an unwillingness by governments <u>and</u> most PPAs to over-refine curricula recommendations to a point where the resulting value-system being promoted would fail to have either majority support or a tenable moral foundation. In spite of the historical progress made by PPAs and their governments in securing basic planned parenthood services, there appears to be a drift to inertia on this subject. The <u>lack</u> of specificity in PPA recommendations to governments within this study testify to this:

the Government should consider providing education for adolescents and adults alike relating to sex roles and

- 254 -

family life . . . to counteract inequalities in the provision of sex/family life education'.(Belgium p. 160)

'Regarding sex education, the de jure situation is satisfactory. However, it is necessary to ensure that reactionary school teachers do not restrict the teaching of the full sex education curriculum in secondary schools. It is also necessary to publish better educational materials both for teachers to use with their pupils and to ecucate teachers themselves. Sexuality, sex education and family planning must be subjects of public consensus rather than confrontation, subject to open debate, where individual convictions and differences in attitude can be taken into account.'.(Poland p. 203)

Given the control of curriculum by individual schools (rather than by government policy) in Britain it is difficult to recommend realistic action by Government.'(UK pg 236).

The problem of limitations on the lengths to which a sympathetic government may go in support of its national PPA is exacerbated in times when an elected government is less sympathetic to the general philosophy of the PPA. Thus the issue of PPA reaction during periods in which it is under threat or attack from right-wing pressure groups which have the sympathy of governments was discussed. This problem is made more complex where PPAs receive government funding.

The UKFPA had experienced a situation in which there had been interference from government over the educational materials which the Association sold and therefore indirectly promoted. At that time, the decision for the Association was whether to reject this interference and risk incurring Parliamentary controversy which may have threatened continued funding, or concede in the short-term to government (or more accurately the right-wing pressure group to which the government was responding). It was decided that to refuse a government 'request' to delete offending sex education materials at this time could not be justified in view of the consequences for the larger part of the Association's work.

It was agreed that PPAs must appreciate and adjust to the political mood of the society if they were to remain a

strong social force with wide political and lay support;
that they must accept the principle that it is the right of
a democratically-elected government to decide the character
of the planned parenthood work it is funding.
Nevertheless, the choice remains with the PPA whether to
work with or without its government. The price to be paid
by a PPA standing against its government may be a loss of
influence through removal of financial power. There was
general agreement that the PPA must never give way on basic
principles, but instead search for initiatives most suited
to the political complexion of the government in power;
that is to say, that there are more options than working
with or without governments. The PPA of the Federal
Republic of Germany has managed to retain funding from a
relatively unsympathetic government while remaining
critical of this government. This has been achieved by
offering the government services which are unobtainable
elsewhere (e.g. abortion counselling to augment the state
abortion services), and purposely avoiding promoting the
more controversial part of the PPA's work (e.g. requesting
funds to assist homosexuals requiring counselling) while
this government is in power. As a line of defence against
the possibility of withdrawal of government support, it is
advisable for PPAs to retain a source of independent income
through commercial sales of its educational materials and
services.

**2. On the subject of sex education/family life education,
the study findings have revealed that most governments are
reluctant to recognise, let alone promote, the <u>right</u> of
young people to information and education to act
responsibly in their nascent sexual lives. In what ways is
it possible for PPAs to work with governments to overcome
the ideological and practical impasse in this area?**

It may be argued that adolescents are likely to accept
responsibility for their sexual behaviour only if certain
rights in this area are implicitly or explicitly
recognised. However, the socialisation of adult
power-holders generally inhibits a willing concession of
rights to the young within cultures in which many taboos
remain attached to sexual expression. Sexual activity is
regarded in the majority of European cultures as properly
the domain of adults. Young (unmarried) people (e.g. up to
18 years) are felt to be transgressing basic norms of

society in enjoying their sexual powers, and potentially
damaging their physical/psychological health and maturation
in doing so. This stance can partially be sustained on
scientific grounds, though the controversy revolves
essentially around that of morality and the threat to
parental authority. Consequently it was agreed that there
is little merit in a PPA appealing to government to further
develop sex education for young people with any other
rationale than the need to forestall their sexual debut on
grounds of health/welfare costs not only to young people
themselves <u>but also to the society in which they live.</u>

While politicians may indeed be sympathetic to the
problems which young people face, governmental interest in
the field of sex education will be secured only if it can
be shown that the state has something <u>tangible</u> to gain from
imparting such information (viz. a saving in health
costs). Of course, governments may also be impelled to act
in reaction to a political pressure group 'threat' either
from their supporters or opponents. The PPA must therefore
tailor its appeal for action accordingly, viz: by focussing
upon health risks rather than social rights. It must also
recognise that in certain political climates its own
ideological stance, or that attributed to it (not all PPAs
choose to present an ideology), will be out of favour.
This fact confirms the necessity of cultivating allies from
opposing political parties who agree with its basic
principles. Of course, the costs of this political
negotiation may be to lose some credibility with the
younger generation itself.

3. What is the function of legislation in furthering planned parenthood rights? To what extent have European laws been influenced by population policies?

The French experience has suggested that it is not
always useful to press for legislation with the intention
of confirming/enforcing individual rights in planned
parenthood because the legal compromise necessary to
achieve such law may create restrictions on access to
services which had not existed previously. Thus, should a
right-wing government come to power in France, the
unsatisfactory abortion law achieved with much struggle in
the 1970s would be enforced restrictively.

The Portuguese experience of recent wide-ranging
legislation in planned parenthood has shown that the law is

of limited value in changing behaviour in the face of the wider socio-cultural process, which can only be influenced by mass education. Thus, it would be unwise to draw any theoretical connection between law and human rights.

Governments are unwilling to espouse population policies as such, preferring to use such euphemisms as health policy, family policy, or 'development' policy aimed at promoting living conditions. Those countries which openly promote population 'planning', such as Yugoslavia, prefer to discuss family planning within the context of women's rights. In any event it was seen to be the role of the PPA to have no part in the direct formulation of a population policy, but to react to government initiatives and monitor their manifest impact and latent consequences.

This role is exemplified in the reaction of Pro Familia, the PPA of the Federal Republic of Germany, to a fund set up by the government (DM 50 million per annum) to provide financial incentives to women to give birth rather than resort to abortion where a pregnancy is unwanted. Pro Familia has calculated that allowances from this fund are inadequate to prevent women taking advantage of it to avoid financial hardship by having a child. On these and other grounds the PPA has publicly challenged the government strategy to increase the population in this way.

In Portugal, the PPA believes that part of its responsibility is to challenge any government economic measure related to the problem of unemployment which may force women to return to the home. This would be regarded as an unacceptable covert population policy.

From the point of view of governments it was noted that no single policy but rather a complex of social policies influence populations, even in contradictory ways. Consequently, it was agreed that one route by which a PPA may influence government is for the former to investigate and report to government latent or unintended consequences to planned parenthood/population of social policies in indirectly related areas such as housing or medical care.

The PPA in the UK sees 4 dimensions to its work: to promote the human right to control fertility; to identify health indicators and call for appropriate action to benefit general health; to promote the welfare of families; and to raise domestic public consciousness of the population, and the world economy. Thus it has campaigned persistently for appropriate contraceptive/educational services to eliminate most of the 200,000 unplanned pregnancies in the UK, a large part of which affect the age group 16-25 at great expense to the health and welfare services. This campaigning is based on long-term targets which are adjusted to suit changes in government, using statistical analyses to substantiate scientifically the economic benefits to be gained.

Conclusion

Summary

M Kozakiewicz

The Dubrovnik seminar has provided a rare opportunity for professionals involved in governments and PPAs to exchange opinions and experiences on most aspects of planned parenthood. Observing the spectrum of local national situations and their political structures, it is possible to identify a simplified but comprehensive typology:

- Federal structure
- Multi-party system
- One-party system

These political structures contain different educational systems, from very centralised operations with centrally-elaborated curricula and a unified programme of teacher-training to fully decentralised systems without a single programme directive. There are structures in which the local governmental level dictates the type of education given, compared with local political structures which are merely organs of central government. These factors influence the type of relationship which can exist between the PPA and government (ministries). The following are 'ideal-types':

- __Adversary__: For example the situation obtaining in Ireland (and which formerly obtained in Portugal and Italy).
- __Partner__: This describes a situation where neither PPA nor government forego their separate identities and differences but choose to cooperate in an agreed area to achieve specific goals (even though these goals may not be concretely specified in advance). This relationship does not exclude non-agreed actions on certain issues, leaving open the possibility of oppositional stances.
- __Ally__: This relationship has a military connotation where the PPA and government share responsibility in dealing with some common objective, organising a division of labour on means and goals.
- __Agent__: Here the PPA is nothing but an executor of government policies, with the latter providing the goals and the means. The PPA is not truly independent (as in the case of some Socialist countries).

Conclusion

In reality, practical examples are likely to share features of more than one type:

- Certain government objectives regarded by the PPA as forms of an unacceptable population policy may be <u>opposed</u>, especially if these aim to restrict free choice/human rights.

- At the same time, the PPA and government may be <u>partners</u> on the subject of implementing recommendations on school sex education, and challenging conservative resistance in these institutions. This may operate as a <u>strategic</u> division of labour, where the PPA, rather than the government itself, agrees to present a challenge to the quality of sex education given in such schools.

- An <u>alliance</u> may be formed between PPA and government on specific issues, such as combatting teenage pregnancies, even though they may be in opposition over general principles.

- The PPA may act as an <u>agent</u> of the government where the latter is simply unable/unqualified to provide certain services to the public (e.g. certain counselling services); the government may use a PPA in this way to fulfil tasks which the government cannot undertake for administrative or political reasons.

A PPA must endeavour to form contacts both with the government in power and with antagonistic political forces (and individuals within such structures who may differ in their opinions). The roles which PPAs can offer include that of:

- <u>Pressure group</u>: This may be welcomed not only by the oppositional party but the government itself, which may find a challenge useful to its own purposes vis-à-vis the media, electorate etc.

- <u>Data bank/research service</u>: The government may welcome the resource as contributing to social policy design. The PPA can also initiate academic research.

- <u>Testing service</u>: PPAs should be workshops in which experiments are forged; they can be known as the innovators of experimental programmes, services, manuals, audio-visuals, media promotions etc., in family planning, sex education, infertility treatment, counselling etc.

Conclusion

PPAs should be discriminatory in their reactions to opponents of planned parenthood. Firstly, there is a wide diversity of opposition reactions - from the extremely aggressive to the moderate; and, secondly, because there is a wide range of individuals within any opposition, some of whom may be cooperative in making compromises. In spite of ideological differences between PPAs and other pressure groups, there are some areas of common interest which may be foci for temporary alliances. For example:

- the desire to eradicate teenage pregnancy (even though some approaches may be discriminatory or unrealistic);
- the desire to limit resort to abortion as a means of planned parenthood (even though some approaches would limit the right to choose in this area);
- the desire to increase moral responsibility for sexual life and its consequences (even though the means to achieve this may differ);
- the desire to increase peoples' awareness of their duty to regulate their fertility (even if by natural methods only).

PPAs should seek to form relations with as many allies as possible, with organisations of: parents, physicians, young people etc., despite the fact that such alliances may be formed around selected issues.

COUNCIL OF EUROPE
COMMITTEE OF MINISTERS

Resolution (75) 29

ON LEGISLATION RELATING TO FERTILITY
AND FAMILY PLANNING(1)

(Adopted by the Committee of Ministers on 14 November 1975
at the 250th Meeting of the Ministers' Deputies)

The Committee of Ministers,

1   Having regard to Recommendation No 2 of the 2nd
European Population Conference on certain social and
economic aspects of fertility trends in Europe, and to the
studies carried out and conclusions put forward by its
Committeee of Demographic Experts;

2   Noting that Resolution 2436 (XXIII) of the General
Assembly of the United Nations refers to "the right of
parents to decide freely and responsibly on the number and
spacing of their children";

3   Noting that the World Population Plan of Action
adopted by the World Population Conference held in
Bucharest in August 1974 affirms that all couples and
individuals have the right to decide freely and responsibly
the number and spacing of their children;

4   Noting further that in the programme of Concerted
International Action for Advancement of Women (1970), the
General Assembly of the United Nations declared one of the
minimum targets of the second United Nations Development
Decade to be the making available to all persons who so
desire of the necessary information and advice to enable
them to exercise that right;

5   Noting the difference in legislation pertaining to
contraception, abortion and economic and social aid to

families in member states, and noting also the marked differences between the de jure and de facto situations which frequently exist in this field;

6   Noting that these differences may lead to social injustice;

7   Noting that the recent decline in fertility in nearly all developed countries has occurred despite these differences in legislation and in its application;

8   Conscious that legislation affecting family planning and aid to families should be seen primarily as a means of allowing people to exercise their discretion.

Recommends member governments:

I   i when formulating policies relating to population to have full regard to the rights and needs of families;
         ii to enable all persons who so desire to have the information and means to decide freely and responsibly on the number and spacing of their children;

II   in order to realise these objectives, to take the following legislative and administrative measures:

A. Family planning services

To make family planning information, advice and means available to all sections of the population as an integral part of health and social services, by means of:

i.   increasing the range and efficiency of family planning services, and ensuring that they are well distributed geographically so as to be within easy reach of the whole population; in this context, special attention needs to be paid to rural areas and the socially disadvantaged areas of large cities;

ii   supporting, where appropriate, the work of non-governmental family planning organisations; this should not be seen as a substitute for action by governments, but should play a clearly defined role in the overall national family planning structure, such organisations being encouraged to continue their work in association with the public health service;

iii   creating where necessary, a national authority or system of co-ordination for action concerning family planning;

iv   taking all necessary steps to publicise family planning services, with the aim of ensuring that all sections of the poulation are fully informed of the facilities to which they are entitled;

v   authorising the supervised advertisement of contraceptives and their distribution after officially approved technical and clinical testing;

vi   ensuring that family planning consultation and the provision of all contraceptives requiring medical supervision are organised in such a way that all income groups may have equal access to them;

vii   encouraging the medical profession to play a part in family planning programmes as an important contribution to good standards of family and community health.

B. Education in family planning

To ensure that all people, especially young people, whether married or single, are informed about the problems and objectives of family planning and about the relative advantages and disadvantages of the various methods available, and in particular by:

i   ensuring that those who are responsible for school curricula, at appropriate levels, are aware of the importance of education in family planning;

ii   making it possible for all couples, and especially those intending marriage, to be able to take advice and instruction on family planning, and encouraging them to do so;

iii   ensuring that those who are responsible for the curricula of medical schools are aware of the importance of including training in the role of doctors in the family planning services;

iv   training social workers, youth workers and paramedical personnel to provide adequate guidance on family planning.

C. Sterilisation

1   To ensure that persons who desire sterilisation are made fully aware that in the present state of knowledge the operation is generally irreversible.

2   To make sterilisation by surgical procedure available as a medical service.

D. Abortion

1   To reduce the need to resort to abortion, in particular by implementing the measures recommended in the other sections of this resolution.

2   To ensure that all legal abortions are carried out under the best possible medical conditions.

3   To ensure that abortion, in those cases where it is permitted by law, is available as a medical service to all women regardless of their social or economic position.

4   To take all necessary steps to eliminate the practice of illegal abortion with its attendant dangers.

E. Economic and social assistance to families

1   To reconsider current systems and levels of family allowances, as well as their periodical revision, and to assess how far the present structure of priorities in social provision - including the relationship between direct and indirect benefits, e.g. tax relief - is appropriate to present social and family needs.

2   To pay special attention to the specific needs of certain families which are statistically in a minority (single-parent families, families with several children etc.)

3   In framing government housing policy, to take account of the real needs of families, having regard to their varying size and structure.

4   To review the position of working people with direct
family responsibilities, in particular with regard to
maximum possible flexibility of working hours, including
opportunities for part-time work, and by extending
provision of crèches, nursery schools and similar services;

III   to report every four years to the Secretary General
of the Council of Europe on the action they have taken on
this resolution.

(1)   Under Rule 10 of the Rules of Procedure for meetings
of the Ministers' Deputies, when it was adopted:
    -   the Representative of Belgium reserved his
government's right not to comply with the text of paragraph
D of this resolution:
    -   the Representative of the Federal Republic of
Germany reserved his government's right not to comply with
the text of paragraph D of this resolution;
    -   the Representative of Ireland, who had abstained
when the vote was taken, reserved his government's right
not to comply with the text of the resolution as a whole.

I 14.336

Resolution (78) 10

ON FAMILY PLANNING PROGRAMMES

(Adopted by the Committee of Ministers on 3 March 1978 at
the 284th meeting of the Ministers' Deputies)

The Committee of Ministers,

Considering that the aim of the Council of Europe is
to achieve a greater unity between its members and that
this aim may be pursued, inter alia, by the adoption of
common regulations in the social and public health field;

Having regard to the terms of reference given by the
European Public Health Committee concerning "reasons for
the failure of some of the existing family planning
programmes in Council of Europe member states and Finland";

Noting that Resolution 2436 (XXIII) of the General
Assembly of the United Nations refers to the "right of
parents to decide freely and responsibly on the number and
spacing of their children";

Considering family planning as an essential part in
quality of life by accepting sexuality as a value in its
own right, not only in connection with reproduction;

Having regard to Resolution (75) 29 of the Council of
Europe, referring to Resolution 2436 (XXIII) of the General
Assembly of the United Nations, to the World Population
Plan of Action adopted by the World Population Conference
held in Bucharest in August 1974 and to the Programme of
Concerted International Action for Advancement of Women
(1970) of the General Assembly of the United Nations, which
recommends member governments "to enable all persons who so
desire to have the information and means to decide feely
and responsibly on the number and spacing of their
children", and also to make "family planning information,
advice and means available to all sections of the

population as an integral part of health and social services";

Considering access to family planning services as a basic human right for both men and women;

Considering that information and advice about family planning concern spacing of pregnancies and contraception as well as problems of infertility;

Considering that information on family planning involves not only delivering technical or medical advice, but also dealing with questions about sexuality and human relationships, and the psychological, ethical and social aspects of living together;

Recognising that there often exists not only a lack of concern but also a certain reluctant attitude among the medical establishment and personnel where family planning is concerned;

Recognising the failure of certain programmes on family planning as due to various reasons: legal, economic, administrative, social-cultural, religious, psychological or political obstacles as well as to the negative impact of some of the mass media;

Recognising that conditions of public health care, legislation on birth control and attitudes towards family planning in member states vary considerably, and that measures and means of a programme must be adjusted to the existing situation.

Recommends governments of member states:

I   to make it possible for the individual to decide freely and responsibly on the number and spacing of children by providing appropriate information and services on family planning as a part of the social and public health service system;

II   to identify and overcome the specific obstacles to setting up a comprehensive family planning programme that may exist;

III   to envisage the following measures when drawing up a family planning programme:

A Planning and management of a family planning programme

i   analyse the needs and demands of the population and define the objectives, the working conditions and the limitations of the programme;

ii   analyse the problems to be solved and the obstacles that may arise;

iii   draw up a plan of action, including a monitoring system with continuous feedback and evaluation;

iv   involve programme personnel and other people concerned, in the planning, management and development of the programme.

B Planning and provision of services

i   provide sufficient and easily available services for it to be possible for everyone who so desires to plan their parenthood by means of preventive measures;

ii   analyse existing resources, and the range of services provided in the healath care system and in non-governmental family planning organisations;

iii   analyse and estimate the need for general family planning services, as well as for special services for high-risk groups;

iv   initiate or strengthen co-operation with the social service system, the private health system and with non-governmental organisations for planned parenthood;

v   organise appropriate services within the public health system, preferably integrated in the maternal and child health setting, in the maternity hospitals and, where existing, in primary health services;

vi   provide family planning services to the individual at minimal cost or free of charge on the same basis as ordinary health care;

vii   provide a sufficient number of qualified and
appropriately trained doctors, midwives, and other
personnel;

viii give particular attention to the emotional and
psycho-sexual implications of family planning for both men
and women;

ix   set up special family planning units for
adolescents and provide special services for other groups
with a high risk of unwanted pregnancy (like women after
abortion and childbirth, and immigrants), target groups
(like parents of teenagers, men in general), and also
infertile couples;

x   encourage and authorise the distribution and
sale of contraceptives through new channels and reinforce
standards and criteria for the quality of different
contraceptives.

C Training and education of personnel

i   make health and social professionals on all
levels understand that family planning is a part of general
health care and therefore part of their responsibilities;

ii   in all education and training, emphasise the
psycho-social aspects of family planning and place it in a
context of sexuality and the whole gamut of human
relations;

iii initiate training of teachers in medical social
and nursing schools and integrate education about family
planning in basic education for doctors, nurses and health
and social personnel in general;

iv   provide appropriate training and continuous in-
service training for the family planning team and personnel
in the public health, social and school system involved in
the family planning programme;

v   make every training programme comprehensive,
delivering knowledge and skills about family planning and
about communication between advisers and advised, and
developing awareness of individual attitudes towards

sexuality and family planning.

D Public information and communication

i   make information activities an integral part of every family planning programme and develop and utilise appropriate methods of communication;

ii   provide comprehensive, reliable and factual information for dissemination through the mass media;

iii   reduce resistance, overcome indifference and bring about changes in attitudes and behaviour by an educational approach, with personal communication as the main instrument;

iv   provide information and encourage knowledge and understanding of family planning by appropriate means of communication, among:

- politicians, decision-makers and leaders of opinion,
- personnel of the medical and social network,
- political, religious and other organisations,
- high-risk groups,
- the general public.

E Evaluation

i   define the objectives and decide what criteria of success and failure to apply;

ii   make evaluation a routine and continuous process, to monitor achievement in the light of objectives, to ensure value for money and to help in future planning;

iii   collect the absolute minimum of data necessary for evaluation and give priority to the most basic data;

iv   ensure the confidentiality and anonymity of the information provided;

v   improve communication between data providers, statisticians and decision-makers in order to draw on the experience of all of them in the planning of the programme.

I 16.917

SEMINAR ON PLANNED PARENTHOOD AS A BASIC HUMAN RIGHT, DUBROVNIK/YUGOSLAVIA, 9–11 DECEMBER 1984 PARTICIPANTS LIST

GOVERNMENT   PLANNED PARENTHOOD ASSOCIATION

BELGIUM

Dr Freddy Deven
Belgische Federatie voor
Gezinsplanning en Seksuele
Opvoeding
BRUSSELS

FRANCE

Mme Cecile Goldet   Mme Colette Gallard
Senateur de Paris   Mouvement Français pour le
PARIS   Planning Familial
                                             PARIS

ITALY

Sa Beatrice Ragoni Machiavelli   Senator Tullia Carettoni
(Member of European Parliament)   Unione Italiana Centri di
ROME   Educazione Matrimoniale e
                                             Prematrimonial
                                             MILAN

POLAND

Prof Mikolaj Kozakiewicz
Towarzystwo Rozwoju Rodzin
WARSAW

PORTUGAL

Prof António Correia de Campos   Dr Albino Aroso
Adviser to Ministry of Health   Associacao para o
LISBON   Planeamento da Familia
                                             LISBON

SPAIN

Dra Sagrario Mateu
Servicio de Salud Publica
Sección Salud Materno-Infantil y
 Planificación Familiar
Ministerio de Sanidad
MADRID

Dra Victoria Abril Navarro
Instituto de la Mujer
Ministerio de Cultura
MADRID

UNITED KINGDOM

Ms Margaret Edwards   Mr Alastair Service
Assistant-Secretary   Family Planning Association
Children's Division   LONDON
Department of Health & Social
 Security
LONDON

YUGOSLAVIA

Mrs Mila Djordjic   Mrs Nevenka Petric
(Deputy Minister for Labour,   Family Planning Council
Health and Social Welfare   of Yugoslavia
BELGRADE   BELGRADE

                               PPA Observer:

                               Mrs Danica Sasic
                               Executive Secretary

IPPF EUROPE REGIONAL PRESIDENT   Dr Jürgen Heinrichs
                                     Pro Familia
                                     FRANKFURT/MAIN

IPPF EUROPE REGIONAL BUREAU   Mr Julian Heddy
                                     Dr Philip Meredith
                                     Ms Lyn Thomas

Issue	De Jure	De Facto
1. Government recognition of human right to number and spacing of children (planned parenthood)	The right of an individual to free determination of the number and spacing of children is not legally regulated in the form of a specific law. This right is nonetheless implied under the adoption by the Government of the International Convention for the protection of human rights and fundamental freedoms.	The Government tends towards a pronatalist position. Consequently, family planning facilities and services are not provided through the state. Sterilisation and abortion services are provided by the state on strict medical criteria.
Protection of family and child	There is a variety of legislation relating to the protection of family and child, under the supervision of the Government welfare department.	
2. Government and other family planning (fp) facilities/services	There is no legislation covering Government family planning facilities, with the exception of female sterilisation.	Government family planning services do not exist. Such services are private, fee-paying, predominantly through gynaecologists' clinics, and through the PPA.
3. The sale, distribution and advertisement of contraceptives	There is no legal regulation governing the sale and advertisement of contraceptives. All contraceptives are permitted to be sold through pharmacies. In the case of orals, which are regarded as medicines, they are subject to the Drugs Act, and must be obtained through a physician's prescription. Provision of all contraceptives through family planning clinics is permitted. Advertising of contraceptives is also permitted.	All contraceptives are sold in pharmacies. Orals are sold in pharmacies on prescription only. Contraceptives are also provided through family planning centres at very low cost. In general, advertising of contraceptives appears mainly in professional literature and magazines.
4. Availability/sale of family planning (fp) related literature	The availability of family planning literature is not legally-regulated. Therefore, the Cyprus PPA meets with no restrictions in providing family planning literature.	Family planning literature is provided only through the Cyprus PPA clinics, and to the public in special information campaigns. The same literature is given to private GPs to display in their waiting rooms. Neither the Government nor any other organisations produce such literature.

*Cyprus joined the Europe Region of the IPPF in 1984

Issue	De Jure	De Facto
5. Sterilisation	Sterilisation is provided for through the Government health services and is legally regulated to the extent that in the case of a married couple both spouses must sign a consent form	Sterilisation is performed in public hospitals though on a rather small scale, and mostly on medical rather than purely family planning grounds. It is also performed by private physicians at high cost as a family planning method. The Cyprus PPA does not provide this service. It is principally a woman's operation, vasectomy being almost unknown.
6. Abortion	Before 1974, abortion was illegal. With the Turkish invasion and the high number of rape victims, the Cyprus PPA campaigned to have abortion legalised. Since this time the regulations covering abortion have been relaxed; amended as follows: 'The basic law (cap 154, SS 167, 168, 169) has been amended by S.4 of Law 59/74 through the addition immediately after S.169 of the following new section:	Abortion, though legally regulated, is widely performed on demand by the private medical sector at high charges. In public hospitals, abortions are performed free of charge on a very small scale and for medical reasons only. In view of the legal situation no statistics are available but it is believed that the rate is reasonably high, including teenage girls.
	S.169 A: Notwithstanding the provision of sections 167, 168, and 169, no person shall be deemed guilty of the offences therein prescribed whenever the pregnancy is terminated under the following circumstances:	
	a)by a medical practitioner duly registered according to the provision of the Medical Practitioners (Registration) Law;	
	b)following a certificate from the appropriate police authority supported by a medical certificate whenever this is possible, that the pregnancy was caused by rape and under circumstances whereby, if the pregnancy was not terminated, serious breakdown would be caused to the social position of the pregnant woman or to her family environment;	
	c)following the bona fide opinion of two medical practitioners, duly registered, that if the pregnancy continued the life of the pregnant woman would be endangered or she or any member of her family would suffer mental or psychological harm, greater than the non-termination of pregnancy or that there exists a real danger that the child, if born, would suffer from serious physical or mental malformation.	

Issue	De Jure	De Facto
7. Infertility treatment	There is no legal regulation covering infertility treatment and artificial insemination.	The Government medical services provide limited facilities for infertility treatment and none for artificial insemination. Only certain private gynaecologists provide such services at very high costs. Although no statistics are available, the infertility rate is believed to be high. Some seek medical advice abroad. The family planning clinics offer infertility referral services.
8. Sex education/family life education	There is no legal provision covering sex education in schools.	Sex education is not included in the school curricula. The Cyprus PPA is the only provider of such education to a wide range of audiences during out-of-school hours. In public high schools, certain sex education elements are incorporated into other subjects such as biology and home economics. The non-inclusion of sex education in the school curricula by the Government is based on moral-ethical grounds. The Cyprus PPA has pioneered the dissemination of sex education materials since 1972 when a campaign was begun to provide sex education to parents, children and youth through out-of-school meetings.
9. Adoption	Adoption is legally regulated. The adoption service operates under the supervision of the Government welfare department. The demands on the potential adoptive parents are defined very strictly. The adoptive parents initially must go through a trial period under the supervision of a welfare officer.	Adoption services are provided only through the Government welfare department. No private organisation exists for providing such services. There are too few children to satisfy demand. In certain cases adoption is carried out through the private adoptive services from Greece.

BIBLIOGRAPHY

Allen, I. Family Planning, Abortion and Sterilisation Services, 1981 Policy Studies Institute, London.

Benn, R. and Peters, S. Social Principles and the Democratic State 1959 George, Allen & Unwin, London.

Berckmans, P. e.a., Adoptie. Een rechtssociologische benadering. 1981 A'pen/ A'dam, De Sikkel/De Ned. Boekhandel

Brodie, E.B. 'Reproductive Freedom, Coercion and Justice' Social Science and Medicine, 1976 Vol 10.

Ceterchi, I. et al, Law and Population Growth in Romania 1974 Bucharest.

Chesnais, J-C. Fertility and the State 1982 European Population Conference EPC (82) 14-E Strasbourg.

Claeys, P-H & Loeb-Mayer, N. Les partis devant le probleme de l'avortement. 1982, Crisp, Bruxelles (CH nr 962)

Coene, M.(red) Statuut van het kind 1980 Brussel, Ced-Samson.

Cossey, D. Abortion and Conscientious Objection 1983 Birth Control Campaign, London.

Coulon, F. 'Les centres de planning familial en Belgique', Cedif Info, 1981, No. 6

Department of Education and Science The School Curriculum 1981 Her Majesty's Stationery Office, London.

Dille-Lobe, V. 'Korte geschiedenis van de gezinsplanning in Belgie', Social Standpunten 1966.

Eversley, D. and Köllmann, W. ed. Population Change and Social Planning 1982 Arnold, London.

GACEHPA, La pratique de l'avortement en Belgique. Etude statistique commentee. 1981 Bruxelles, Octobre.

Hindell, D. & Simms, M. Abortion Law Reformed 1971 Peter Owen

Johnson, T. Postcoital Contraception 1982 Pregnancy Advisory Services, London.

Leathard, A. The Fight for Family Planning 1980 Macmillan, London.

Lesthaeghe, R. The Decline of Belgian Fertility, 1800-1970 1977 Princeton University Press.

Lesthaeghe, R. 'A Century of Demographic and Cultural Change in Western Europe: an Exploration of Underlying Dimensions' in Population and Development Review 1983 9, 3.

Ministerie van Volksgezondheid en van het Gezin. Bewustouderschap. Bericht over informatieverspreiding. (Dutch version) 1977 Brussel, Dienst Pers & Voorlichting, Ministerie van Volksgezondheid. Jaarverslagen.

Marques-Pereira, B. L'interruption volontaire de grossesse: un processus de politisation I+II. 1981 Crisp, Bruxelles (CH nr 923 CH nr 930-931).

McIntosh, C.A. Population Policy in Western Europe 1983 M E Sharpe Inc.

Meredith P. Pharmacy, Contraception and the Health Care Role 1982 FPA, London.

Ministerie van Justitie. Enige beschouwingen over het abortusvraagstuk. (Dutch version) 1972 Brussel.

National Swedish Board of Education Instruction Concerning Interpersonal Relations 1977 Liber Utbildningsförlaget, Stockholm.

Pauwels, J.M. Recht inzake seksualitiet 1982 (2) Uitg. Acco. Leuven.

Rifflet, M. 'Le controle des naissances en Belgique', La Nouvelle Revue, 1973, 29e annee, 1.

Simons, J. Fertility Control in Europe, European Population Conference 1982, EPC(82) 3-E Strasbourg.

Smith, W. Campaigning for Choice, 1978 FPA.

Steadman-Jones G. Outcast London Peregrine London 1971.

Stengers, J. 'Les pratiques anticonceptionelles dans le marriage au XIXe siècles: problèmes humains et attitudes religieuses' in Révue Belge de Philosophie et d'Histoire 1971, 49.

Suitters, B. Be Brave and Angry 1973 IPPF.

Van de Kaa, D.J. 'Towards a Population Policy for Western Europe' in Population Decline in Europe, 1978 Council of Europe.

Van den Brekel, J C. Population Policy in the Council of Europe: Policy Responses to Low Fertility Conditions, European Population Conference 1982, EPC (82) 15-E Strasbourg.

Van Look, M. Evolutie van het Belgisch adoptierecht. T Privaatrecht, 1970, (4).

Van Praag, Ph. 'De opkomst van het nieuw-malthusianisme in Vlaanderen' in T. Soc. Geschied. 1977.

Willems, P. Wijewickrema, S. & Lesthaeghe, R. 'De evolutie van de bruchtbaarheid in Belgi, 1950-1980', Bevolking & Gezin, 1981, 3.

Willems, P. et al.,'De evolutie van de vruchtbaarheid in Belgie, 1950-80' in Bevolking & Gezin 1981, 3.

Willems, P. & Wijewickrema, S. 'De evolutie van de nuptialitiet van 1954 tot 1981 Bevolking & Gezin, 1984, 3 (in druk).

Willems, P. & Wijewickrema, S. 'De evolutie van de

nuptialiteit van 1954 tot 1981' in <u>Bevolking & Gezin</u> 1984.
Yuan Tien, H. 'Changing population policy approaches in
China', <u>Intercom</u> 1981 Vol 9, No 10.

INDEX